THE DMSO HANDBOOK

A New Paradigm in Healthcare

Hartmut P. A. Fischer

THE DMSO HANDBOOK

A NEW PARADIGM IN HEALTHCARE

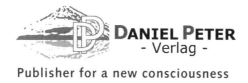

DANIEL PETER
- Verlag -

Publisher for a new consciousness

Copyright	© 2015 Daniel-Peter-Verlag, Schnaittach

Publisher	Daniel-Peter-Verlag, Schnaittach
Email	*info@daniel-peter-verlag.de*
Internet	www.daniel-peter-verlag.de
Translation from the German	Dr Seiriol Dafydd
Editing / proofreading	Dr Rhiannon Ifans
Cover design	Frank Alkemade, Alkemade Fotografie photo under license from kikkerdirk© – fotolia.com
Layout and typesetting	Hans-Jürgen Maurer, Frankfurt am Main
ISBN	978-3-9815255-5-7

Translated from the third German edition.

ACKNOWLEDGEMENTS

A number of wonderful people have made it possible for this book to be completed; some of them are not even aware of how they have helped. A friendly conversation, or assistance with other tasks can, directly or indirectly, help to bring a project forward. One does not always recall these numerous moments and therefore the following list is certainly not comprehensive.

Thank you:

Dr Antje Oswald, who trustingly placed this project in my hands.

My family, for their support and understanding as I was working on this book; in particular my wife, who patiently advised and corrected despite having an engineering company of her own to manage.

Dr Marco Fuß, who unearthed the results of a number of DMSO studies.

My PhD supervisor, *Professor Manfred Christl,* whose admirable breadth of knowledge inspired many ideas.

All my colleagues, fellow health practitioners and doctors who, through open exchanges of knowledge and experience, contributed a number of additions, case experiences and new ideas.

My patients and students, who made an important contribution through conducting their numerous self-experiments, and writing experience reports.

Udo Bauch, whose experience provided me with a number of treatment suggestions. He was a victim of the Eschede train crash on 3 June 1998 and has since published a book describing his personal story.

Mr G., whose 'DMSO cases' were an important stimulus. His lateral thinking and unconventional approach to life's big topics have been an inspiration, raising justified questions regarding commonly-held assumptions.

Our dear assistants *Helga and Udo Gerstendorff,* whose professional and life experience provided important impetus.

My former schoolteacher *Dr Rainer Ganns*, who inspired in me an everlasting interest in science.

CONTENTS

«YOUR HEALTH IS OUR MISSION!»

FOREWORD

Having been treasured as a secret for many years by just a small number of specialists and alternative practitioners, DMSO is currently enjoying a remarkable comeback in the field of alternative medicine. It has mainly become known as a fast-acting, well-tolerated treatment for acute inflammations and for traumatic injuries. It has an anti-inflammatory effect, relieves pain immediately, accelerates the swift resorption of swellings and haemorrhages, and supports wound healing. It is a very popular treatment for sports injuries, shoulder–arm syndrome, rheumatic and degenerative joint disease (including degenerative changes in the intervertebral discs) and neuralgia. However, DMSO can do much more than that. It is not only cosmetic surgeons, A&E doctors, sports therapists and veterinarians who have discovered its advantages, but also countless lay people who were searching for an alternative cure for chronic pain. This natural substance is an extremely useful basis for therapeutic self-reliance, and is a huge leap towards freedom from the many side effects caused by standard medications. Until this time, patients searching for a solution to their problems have not had access to information concerning this medication's fields of application, or to clear instructions concerning its safe use. There has, surprisingly, been no comprehensive reference handbook outlining the practicalities of using this wonderful substance. This book is therefore intended as a practical, application-oriented reference book for patients who treat themselves, as well as for doctors, alternative health practitioners and other therapists.

Last October, Dr Antje Oswald was asked by the publisher to write this book and she passed on that request to me. After initial discussions with Daniel Peter, I could never have imagined the consequences of agreeing to take on the project – in the most positive sense. Now, all the discoveries and eureka moments, all the marvelling and the astonishment at the research done on this substance since it was first presented to the world 146 years ago, are here in print – ripe for application in treating a wide variety of illnesses. I have used DMSO both personally and professionally to treat a range of conditions and you can now draw upon this experience without having to reinvent the wheel each time.

I have been familiar with and have used DMSO for a very long while. The substance – a solvent with exceptional properties – was a constant companion during my scientific studies, and as I carried out the research for my dissertation in the field of organic synthesis. It is used in chemical reactions as well as in analytic tests in the field of nuclear magnetic resonance spectroscopy, for example. After undergoing a special activation process it can even be used as a mild oxidiser (Swern oxidation). However, its widespread use as a liquid component for solutions in research and industry is only one display, one aspect, of DMSO.

The true value of DMSO as a treatment for various conditions in both humans and animals was first revealed in the early 1960s through experiments conducted on transplant tissue and carried out by Stanley W. Jacob M.D. in Oregon. Since then he has been regarded, alongside Edward E. Rosenbaum M.D., as the father of the medicinal use of DMSO, which has since then experienced an unpredictable and fluctuating history. The story has been vividly recounted by Maya Muir in a survey article:[1] it has moved from suddenly being championed as a miracle cure by big pharmaceutical companies who made approval applications for its use[*], to becoming the well-kept secret of a community of holistic health practitioners; from being an object of covetousness to which tens of thousands of scientific research papers have been devoted, to becoming an obscure medicine used by wealthy patients in Central American countries, where it is officially approved for medicinal use.

Even though a vast number of scientific papers have been published on the therapeutic use of DMSO, and even though the bulk and quality of the data gathered regarding cured patients is unmatched by any other alternative treatment, until now there has, surprisingly, been no comprehensive reference handbook for therapists and patients. Many people are familiar only with its name, 'DMSO', and with its main fields of application, but because instructions and formulas have generally been hard to come by, and because these have often been jealously guarded by those in the know, a certain insecurity has developed with regard to the use of this extremely versatile substance. That is why this book is intended first and foremost as a practical guide to the safe use of DMSO. Having said that, I hope this book can also be regarded as an engaging

---

[*] News: As of November 2015 DMSO ampules are officially available in Germany!

and stimulating read since many sections go beyond what is, strictly speaking, the DMSO horizon, giving you a good deal of information on related fields.

As a scientist I could not help but begin the book with a chapter that covers DMSO's interesting history, its astonishing physical, chemical and pharmacological properties, as well as its safety as a natural medicine. For the more impatient readers, which I suspect includes not only medical lay persons but also some doctors and alternative practitioners, short summaries have been included **at the beginning** of these sections. This will enable you to avoid the more detailed information on the characteristics of DMSO and to move on to the practical chapters quickly. However, I highly recommend that you return later to read the scientific sections. Doing so will give you a deeper understanding of the biochemical processes in humans and animals that DMSO gives rise to. It may also help you to reconcile and build your own personal link between theory and practical application.

The greater part of this book is dedicated to practical application techniques and administration methods, as well as to the various symptoms and illnesses that can be successfully treated using DMSO. This is a reference book that teaches the safe use of DMSO, encourages you to try it for yourself, and makes it possible for you to become familiar with this mysterious, healing substance.

Due to sheer habit, this book is sprinkled with little digs, or even substantiated accusations, against doctors and orthodox medicine. Judge for yourself whether these are justified and I ask for leniency. Relations between doctors and alternative practitioners are polarised – that is the way it has always been. These days, however, orthodox physicians attend my seminars with the result that friendly and trusted networks are formed across professional boundaries. Inversely, I too need the assistance of doctors. Not only when I fracture a bone, but also when it comes to diagnosis reports, or pharmacological assessments. It is perfectly clear to me, as it should be to all alternative practitioners, that doctors, due to their extensive, structured training programmes, are usually far ahead of us in terms of specialist medical knowledge, and in their experience of treating patients. They can also offer holistic, well-tolerated treatments that are focused on the individual. Unfortunately they are hindered by the close, triangular bond that exists between the medical insurance authorities (or the NHS in the UK), the pharmaceutical and medical technology companies, and the bodies that represent doctors' own interests. Many doctors start their careers in the healing profession highly motivated and full of ideals, only to become resigned to the fact that monetary limitations and bureaucracy rob them of their professional freedom. To make matters worse, many doctors adopt the studied arrogance of the university professors and hospital bosses with regard to learning new things and admitting mistakes. It would do them good to open their minds to alternative and unpatented medicines such as DMSO, and all the other alternatives mentioned in this book. Those who take a categorical stand against everything the pharmaceutical industry tries to suppress, and who thereby directly or indirectly sell themselves out to this industry, are needlessly throwing away an opportunity to see beyond the limitations of their own profession. Would it not be excellent to view a generation of doctors, therapists and alternative practitioners working together, using all freely available, effective and well-tolerated medications for the good of the patient? When we look at those who are not motivated by money, we see that both factions are already making an equally valuable contribution to public health – and this is something that should be acknowledged and appreciated by all.

Hartmut Fischer

INTRODUCTION

DMSO is well known as an easy-to-use remedy that is just as suitable for serious and extremely painful illnesses as it is for day-to-day complaints. It can be used with excellent results and there is no need to fear any undesired adverse effects. So far, findings suggest that DMSO can be combined with other remedies to great effect, and that it can amplify the influence of other substances. DMSO is widely available and very affordable. So if you came across this book while searching for a solution to your individual health problems, or while searching for a therapeutic approach to assist patients, it is worth examining DMSO and all its remarkable characteristics more closely. Since the safety of any treatment should be your primary concern, I would at this point like to briefly mention the few accompanying effects of DMSO treatment. Not all users experience these.

We could have long discussions about what should be regarded as a side effect and how that might be distinguished from the desired effect. In this book, phenomena that occur due to the application of a medical substance are always regarded as desired and necessary if they are an expression of the hoped-for pharmacological effect on the organism. This is irrespective of whether the individual user subjectively appraises that effect as being pleasant or unpleasant, because, after all, an effect was desired. For example, when applied externally DMSO opens the capillaries; this leads to a temporary and local redness of skin, which can vary greatly from individual to individual (see Chapter 2.2). Since this reaction helps to significantly accelerate the alleviation of swelling, and the healing of acute injuries, I naturally regard it as part and parcel of the desired effect. To take a more drastic example: if you take an emetic agent, you would hope and expect the desired effect, which in this case is subjectively very unpleasant, to occur reliably and unfailingly!

In contrast, I regard hair loss when undergoing the orthodox medical treatment of chemotherapy as one example of a (genuine) undesired side effect. This is clearly an unselective, cell-damaging substance; hair loss is an indication that the body's own healthy tissue has been damaged. This is obviously not desirable and need not be accepted as necessary.

Such an interpretation of 'effects and side effects' is in conflict with the current norm in clinical records and questionnaires. The local redness of skin, which quickly abates, would normally be noted under the heading 'Observed Side Effects'. We are very familiar with this dilemma in the field of alternative healing and such phenomena are often described using the term 'initial aggravation'. It is well known that detoxification and purging processes can cause intense and unpleasant adverse effects ranging from nightmares to nausea. However, neither the practitioner nor the patient would speak of undesired side effects in such a context. Firstly, these reactions are expected; they are desired. Secondly, they are not a side effect, but the main effect.

It is likely that one specific characteristic of DMSO will be regarded by some as disadvantageous. In many users DMSO produces a mouth and / or body odour that is described by others as being similar to the smell of garlic or oysters. Funnily enough, the users themselves are not aware of this smell and are often surprised that others keep their distance or open a window. The body's natural excretion processes ensure that this odour disappears at the latest within 72 hours of taking DMSO. This characteristic of DMSO is, incidentally, the main reason why it is difficult if not impossible to conduct double blind trials on the substance. It would be instantly clear which test subjects had been given the verum and which had received the placebo.

Further accompanying effects of external DMSO treatment can include the previously mentioned skin irritations (redness, itching, burning and flaking). These effects are all reversible and vary greatly from individual to individual. It should also be mentioned that it takes time to become accustomed to the taste of DMSO when it is taken as a drink. But again statements by patients, therapists and users vary greatly in this regard. I have heard a range of opinions, from 'very bitter' to 'very pleasant'. Each person is an individual. Because of this taste, some people recommend preparing DMSO using fruit or vegetable juice instead of water. Always carry out a tolerance test before using DMSO as a treatment. This can be done by dabbing a 70% DMSO solution onto the skin at the elbow crease – slight redness, itching or prickling can be regarded as normal. Individuals can also test DMSO using kinesiology, or using bio-resonance.

What we have here, then, is a substance that causes a conspicuous odour in many users, tastes bitter, and triggers various short-term skin reactions when applied externally. Would that stop you from using this substance to heal or alleviate your own or others' suffering? What if I were to tell you that it can even dissolve pathological calcification in the shoulders? Of course, the negative characteristics must be taken into consideration and, during my first few self-experiments, they led me to plan the timing of the application meticulously so as to have as little impact on my private and professional life as possible, and to optimise the duration of application. Compared with these few harmless side effects, the therapeutic possibilities are staggering and extremely valuable. You will not want to miss out on them.

Only once in the history of medicinal DMSO use did speculation arise regarding possible long-term side effects. The (premature) concerns expressed during the period of extensive animal testing studies in the mid-1960s were attributable to the enormously high doses (up to 100 times the recommended daily dose for humans) and were limited to a few laboratory animals. Concerns arose with regard to changes observed in the refractive properties of the lens of the eyes in three species of animals following weeks of high-dose application. Simply put, the rabbits, pigs and dogs[2] became short-sighted after being given high doses of DMSO. This data was used by the lead scientists in The New York Academy of Sciences publication in 1965 and led to the US approval authority, the Food and Drug Administration (FDA), issuing a temporary halt on all clinical studies even before the journal was published.[*] However, the results could not be reproduced later in rabbits when using normal doses, and such effects have never been observed in humans or other higher mammals.[3]

From an ethical and therapeutic perspective there is one drawback to the medicinal use of DMSO, or dimethyl sulfoxide, and that is the fact that it is not widely available within the framework of medical prescriptions because only very few DMSO-based medicinal products are officially approved for human use anywhere in the world. This is obviously linked to the limited patentability of a cheap solvent that is widely available, and to the resistance shown by the approval authorities. The only option left is to take the opportunity of walking this alternative path alone, or with the guidance of a doctor or alternative practi-

---

[*] News: As of November 2015 DMSO ampules are officially available in Germany!

tioner familiar with DMSO use. It is the only option available when officially approved, profitable medications or treatments have long failed to bring about a cure or are too toxic and harmful, thereby forcing people to take health issues into their own hands. This book will help you on that path.

This book's single most important message is: never allow anyone to tell you that your illness is incurable simply because it is chronic or severe. No matter what that illness may be! This mental strength is incredibly important in terms of the decisions you make regarding your treatment, particularly when it comes to making the conscious decision to turn away from counterproductive treatment options as early as possible. Further damage to the immune system, injuries caused by unnecessary operations, and weakness resulting from them, can quickly make an illness life-threatening. In his book *Krebs natürlich heilen* [Curing Cancer Naturally], the biochemist and naturopath Walter Last wonderfully illustrates the correlation between an explicit renunciation of Chemo & Co. and an improved opportunity of being healed using holistic alternative treatments. There is no doubt that it is well worth searching for an individual healing path. In doing so you can disengage yourself from unhelpful patterns, and your body can find its way back to a place where it can function normally, ideally without submitting to the surgeon's knife or to synthetic medications and their many side effects. Ultimately, your body (as well as your mind and spirit) has to heal and regenerate itself. DMSO can be an important stimulus to help make that happen!

You are presumably familiar with some of DMSO's possible applications. But alongside its main use as a treatment for sports injuries, soft tissue / joint problems, and scar healing, it is important that you also discover the huge potential it has in all aspects of tissue regeneration. With this in mind, I want to encourage you to study the following chapter which sets DMSO within its scientific context. Despite the scientific terminology, which is to some extent unavoidable, I have attempted to make these observations as interesting and informative as possible. I am convinced that we all have a natural curiosity to delve more deeply into the 'essentials of life' than day-to-day life usually allows. Approaching the phenomena of health and illness from the perspective of the exact sciences, in contrast to the purely symptom-oriented observations of orthodox medicine, can be extremely helpful to understanding the complex interplay between substances and the body. Ernst Peter Fischer, a well-known science historian, writes with great perspicacity in his book *Die andere Bildung: Was man von den Naturwissenschaften wissen sollte* [A different Education: What you should know about Science]: 'Without knowledge of the basics of and recent developments in the most important sciences, we find it increasingly difficult to grasp the world around us. As responsible citizens we wish to evaluate and decide on the use of biotechnologies, to express our opinion on atomic power or the threat of climate change, we want to be part of the decision-making process as regards setting the course for research, health and education policy. But all too often we lack the basic knowledge required to make responsible decisions in these fields.' In another section he writes: '... our society's lack of education becomes apparent in the fact that scientific theories are measured by the same yardstick as their less developed cousins.'

'Anything that is against nature will not abide for any length of time.'
Charles Darwin

SCIENTIFIC ASPECTS

D MSO is a substance that can be described objectively: its molecules display measurable physical and chemical characteristics. Furthermore, DMSO, once taken by higher animals, also has analysable pharmacological effects that cause various physiological reactions. It is important to determine exactly how safe each substance is – even cooking salt has a toxic threshold. By reading the following sections you will acquire a different perspective on DMSO and its uses. That should give you a sense of security as you make your own therapeutic experiments and as you apply it to treat illnesses that may not be listed here. Most importantly, however, you will learn what DMSO can do and what it cannot do, so that you can make responsible decisions when choosing a treatment.

1.1 WHAT IS DMSO?

Summary

DMSO is the abbreviation of DiMethyl SulfOxide, a transparent, odourless liquid; a natural substance that is obtained from wood. Countless scientific and medical studies have shown that this liquid displays an astonishing range and quality of healing effects in humans and animals.

It can be applied externally onto the skin, or taken internally as a diluted drink or by injection / infusion. In the human body, a very small part of it is broken down into a substance which in most users causes a temporary odour that is described as 'oyster-like'. The vast majority of the DMSO administered, however, is gradually converted in the body to organic sulphur (MSM). This substance has an extremely positive effect on the (connective) tissue and is often used to treat joint problems. DMSO exerts a comprehensive range of effects on the health that includes powerful regeneration, swift balancing action and natural repair.

Viewed submicroscopically, dimethyl sulfoxide is a liquid that is made up of very small individual particles, namely the molecules with the formula C_2H_6SO or $(CH_3)_2SO$ and that has a molecular mass of $M = 78$ grams per mole. As a point of comparison, insulin, a natural hormone that regulates blood sugar levels, has a molecular mass of $M = 5734$ grams per mole, while water has a molecular mass of only 18 grams per mole. The name 'dimethyl sulfoxide' reveals that it is a member of the sulfoxide group of substances, which are characterised by the following structure:

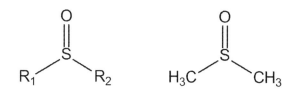

Figure 1: Sulfoxides with arbitrary organic deposits and DMSO

The characteristic structural element here, the S=O group, an oxidised sulphur atom ('sulphur oxide'), is complemented by two arbitrary organic deposits in these molecules. Therefore, DMSO is the simplest symmetrical sulfoxide with two identical methyl groups as further ligands of the central sulphur atoms. So in this case: $R_1 = R_2 = \text{-CH}_3$. DMSO and *Discovery* higher sulfoxides (diethyl sulfoxide, dibutyl sulfoxide, etc.) were first discovered in 1865–66 by the Russian chemist Alexander Mikhaylovich Zaitsev (1841–1910), who originally studied at Kazan University. This is the one and the same Zaitsev (alternative spellings: Zaytsev / Saytzeff / Saytzev) after whom the famous Zaitsev's rule, which predicts the favoured alkene product(s) in elimination reactions, is named. Thanks to the influence of his teacher Alexander Butlerov, Zaitsev spent the years between 1863 and 1870 conducting research alongside some of Western Europe's most important scientists. The work on the various sulfoxides was conducted as part of his doctoral dissertation which he submitted to the German chemist Hermann Kolbe at Leipzig University in 1865. At the same time, he sent his sulfoxide manuscripts and descriptions of other, new compounds to the editorial board of what was then the most important journal in the field, *Liebigs Annalen der Chemie und Pharmazie*, which had been under the editorship of Justus von Liebig and Emanuel Merck since 1832. It was in this journal that Zaitsev's DMSO discovery was first published in 1867.[4]

In that publication Zaitsev writes: 'Dimethyl sulphur oxide is very similar to the oxides I have previously described. It is a thick, colour- and odourless liquid that only solidifies into a crystalline mass when cooled. Even though it becomes somewhat volatile at a temperature of 100 °C, it cannot be distilled without decomposing. It is readily soluble in water, alcohol, and ether. Zinc and diluted sulphuric acid reduce the dimethyl sulphur oxide (back) to dimethyl sulphide.'

Transformation into MSM

The article also describes the further oxidation of DMSO into di- methyl sulfone ($DMSO_2$). This substance is produced when an addi- tional oxygen atom is attached to the central sulphur atom and, like DMSO, it is a widely used treatment that is popularly known as MSM.

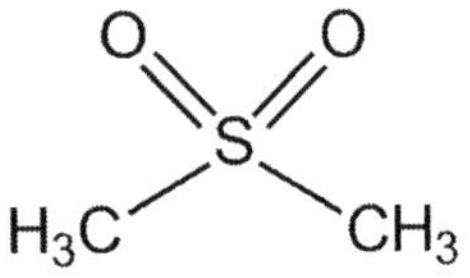

Figure 2: MSM

MSM (methylsulfonylmethane or dimethyl sulfone) is used as an 'or- ganic sulphur' to treat arthrosis. It is also used as a general nutritional supplement to aid connective tissue regeneration and it is widely used in veterinary medicine. Our interest in MSM here concerns its status as the natural decomposition product of DMSO in humans and animals.[5,6,7] To be more precise, it is formed as a metabolite of DMSO when DMSO is oxidised by the well-known cytochrome P450 enzyme system in the liver. As a water-soluble compound it is then excreted via the kidneys – at least that part of the substance that was not otherwise metabolised, as is desired when taking MSM in a targeted manner. After taking DMSO, MSM can be detected in the urine for a significantly longer pe- riod of time than the unchanged DMSO, which is fully excreted within about two days. This has been documented in great detail by Gerhards and Gibian, two researchers at the Berlin company Schering AG, in a 1968 article in the journal *Naturwissenschaften* that is worth reading.[8] So DMSO treatment (fortunately) always supplies the connective tissue with the 'organic sulphur' MSM. It has even been proven that MSM, or to call it by its more scientific name, $DMSO_2$, can be detected in human urine without the intentional delivery of DMSO[9] and is also found in the tissue of other animals. So methylsulfonylmethane is clearly present in the tissue and bodily fluids of higher mammals. Since we could write a whole book about MSM, its effects and its fields of application, we will now return to examine Zaitsev's work more closely.

So we can say that there is an 'oxidation chain' that starts with dimethyl sulphide (DMS) and leads, via DMSO, to methylsulfonylmethane (MSM).

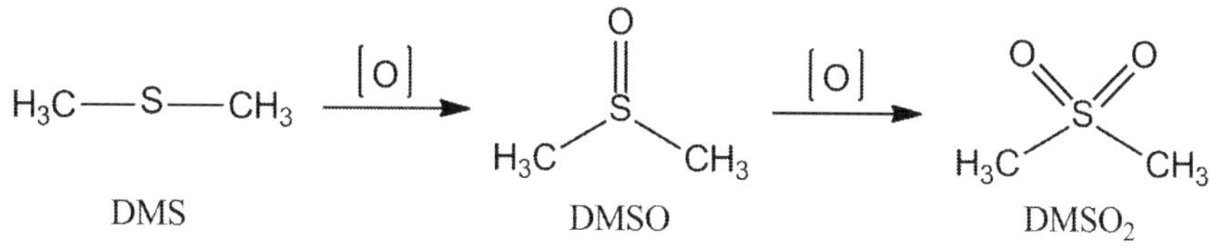

Figure 3: Two-stage oxidation beginning with dimethyl sulphide

In the body, both steps in the oxidative process can be carried out by appropriate enzyme systems. In the laboratory, these steps can be carried out stage by stage through reactions with hydrogen peroxide, potassium permanganate, or nitric acid, as Zaitsev used. These days such processes are not necessary because DMSO is obtained as an industrial by-product from lignin in paper manufacturing.

The reduction of DMSO into dimethyl sulphide (DMS) that occurs on a small scale (about 0.5 to 1.0%[10,11]) in the human body is the physiological cause of the mouth and body odour described above. This happens no matter whether the DMSO is applied to the skin, taken orally or administered intravenously. DMS has a boiling point of exactly 37 °C and is, as a result, expelled from the body mainly via the lungs as a gaseous metabolite, as is the case with carbon dioxide in energy metabolism. Another reason for the odour might be catalysed rearrangements of alkyl disulphides (in this case methyl disulphides), as is common when the alliin in garlic and other plants in the allium genus is metabolised. It is known that these decomposition products and their metabolites are also produced in varying degrees from individual to individual and not everyone perceives them as having an unpleasant odour, although many do.

Characteristic odour

Here is a little anecdote as a brief diversion. Back in the summer of 1995 I had the pleasure of having dinner with Kuno Lichtwer and his wife at a restaurant not far from the headquarters of his company in the Wallenroder Straße in Berlin-Reinickendorf. As background information you should know that he is known as the father of 'garlic therapy'. In the mid-1980s his company, Lichtwer Pharma, was the first pharmaceutical producer of garlic extract tablets (Kwai®, Sapec®), making them socially acceptable and available on prescription. In addition, clinical studies were carried out on his initiative to prove the efficacy of garlic as a treatment for hypertension and elevated blood lipids. This man, who was once called the 'Garlic King' by *Focus* magazine, ordered his meal, asking the waiter for the special of the day but 'without garlic'! He then turned to me and added that it would be good if everyone around our table chose a garlic-free dish. In case you misunderstand me, he did not say that because he is inherently against garlic but because the results of the clinical and pharmacological studies indicate that only garlic extract obtained in a protected atmosphere possesses the desired medicinal effect of alliin and its enzymatic reaction product allicin. He claims that garlic prepared normally during cooking has no beneficial effect on health because of the premature contact with the oxygen in the air. As a result, Mr Lichtwer considers it to be a superfluous annoyance. In hindsight, such talk over dinner could easily be interpreted as a marketing exercise. Everyone who uses garlic when cooking will know that it has a positive effect on their health.

Natural occurrence By now we know that small quantities of both DMSO and MSM are naturally present in many of the foods we eat every day. These foods include milk, tomatoes, tea, coffee, beer and many others. Incidentally, the direct reduction product of naturally occurring DMSO, the 'smelly' dimethyl sulphide, also forms during cooking, for example when preparing seafood and certain types of vegetables.[12] Bacterial metabolic processes in heated plant foods (e.g. when malting) can also lead to the formation of DMS from the amino acid S-Methylmethionine that is present in it. Certain bacteria present in the oral flora can also produce this substance, which can then lead to bad breath without the person having taken DMSO. DMS can also be readily detected in the atmosphere because it is emitted in large quantities by the phytoplankton in the oceans. So perhaps we should simply relax when patients undergoing DMSO treatment breathe out tiny quantities of the stuff.

The section bears the tile 'What is DMSO?'. C. F. Brayton succinctly answers this question in an excellent overview study, which states:[13]

Dimethyl sulfoxide (DMSO) is a very simple compound that has stimulated much controversy in the scientific and popular literature. It is an aprotic solvent. Therapeutic and toxic agents that are not soluble in water are often soluble in DMSO. DMSO has a very strong affinity for water; on exposure to air, pure DMSO is rapidly diluted. DMSO's physiologic and pharmacologic proper ties and effects are incompletely understood. Properties that are considered to be particularly important to its therapeutic and toxic effects include: its own rapid penetration and enhanced penetration of other substances across biologic membranes; free radical scavenging; effects on coagulation; anticholinesterase activity; and DMSO-induced histamine release by mast cells. DMSO's systemic toxicity is considered to be low.

An eternal puzzle

These few lines make it clear that DMSO possesses a wide range of effects and potential fields of application. For this reason DMSO is often not only regarded as a single medication, but it is also used as a comprehensive treatment approach. So let us learn more about this substance so that we can understand its characteristics more thoroughly.

1.2 PROPERTIES

The first description of the substance properties of DMSO compiled by the Russian chemist Alexander Zaitsev (see previous section) appears basic compared with what we know today and much can be added to it. Traditionally, substance descriptions are divided into physical, chemical and pharmaceutical / pharmacological sections. But just as the fixed boundaries between scientific disciplines that have developed over the centuries are becoming increasingly blurred, the various properties of DMSO covered in the following sections are closely intertwined. Both users and scientific researchers will ultimately have to agree that this medicinal substance still retains many secrets and surprises.

1.2.1 Physical properties

Summary

DMSO can be mixed with water in any ratio. Because of this any dilution can be prepared using various kinds of water. When DMSO is left in an open container it even absorbs moisture from the air. It has a bitter taste and, in contrast to water, it 'freezes' when the temperature drops below 18.5 °C. Storage containers should therefore be kept warm, particularly in winter. However, if DMSO solidifies it will return to a liquid state when it is warmed up again. Containers / bottles do not break when DMSO freezes, unlike water which expands as it solidifies. DMSO does not have a tendency to vaporise at normal room and skin temperatures and it does not evaporate when left in open containers or when applied to the skin. DMSO is only marginally heavier than water: 1 litre weighs 1.1kg.

Before proceeding to describe the physical properties of DMSO, below is a table listing its measurable properties.[14,15,16 and others] To make these abstract, purely theoretical values somewhat more meaningful I have, where possible, included the comparable values of water, a liquid we are all very familiar with since we use it every day of our lives, see table 1.

The indication 'odourless' refers to pure DMSO. As soon as small quantities of the reduction product DMS is present, the odour is described as having a garlic- or oyster-like quality.

The term 'hygroscopic' describes the behaviour of substances that show a strong tendency to absorb water. It is well known, for example, that (common) salt that is left out to stand absorbs the moisture in the air and becomes lumpy or even turns into liquid. This effect is used specifically to dehumidify or dry the air, i.e. to dehydrate organic solvents using appropriate hygroscopic salts. If the hygroscopic substance is already in a liquid state, as DMSO is, then water absorption is naturally less pronounced. However, if you leave a defined quantity of it in a measuring cylinder, in open contact with the air, and at a temperature of at least 19 °C, then water absorption can be up to 10% of the original volume. So we should bear in mind that a stock of DMSO that has been left in contact with the air for a long period of time is potentially already a 90% solution and that less water can be added later.

Water absorption

Property	Values for DMSO	Values for water, as a comparison
Appearance / physical state	Clear, colourless and odourless liquid	Clear, colourless and odourless liquid
Water absorption from air (hygroscopic effect)	Up to 10%	–
Solubility	Readily soluble in water, alcohol …	Readily soluble in DMSO
Taste	Bitter	Neutral
Melting point	18.5 °C (292 K)	0 °C (273 K)
Boiling point	189 °C (462 K)	100 °C (373 K)
Density	1104kg·m^{-3} (20 °C)	1000kg·m^{-3} (20 °C)
Vapour pressure	0.56 mbar (20 °C)	23.4 mbar (20 °C)
Molar mass	78.13 g/mol	18.02 g/mol
Viscosity	2.14 mPa·s (20 °C)	1.001 mPa·s (20 °C)
Flash point	87–95 °C (360 K)	Non-flammable
Ignition temperature	300 °C (573 K)	Non-flammable
Dissociation constant (pK$_a$)	35	14
Permittivity	49 AsV^{-1}m^{-1}	81 AsV^{-1}m^{-1}
Thermal capacity	1.97 kJ/kg·K (25 °C)	4.18 kJ/kg·K (20°C)
Dipole moment	4.3 D	1.84 D
Coefficient of thermal expansion	0.00088 K^{-1}	0.21 K^{-1}

Table 1: Selected physical properties of DMSO

There is no limit to how much water you can add when diluting DMSO – both substances can be mixed in any ratio. The practical part of the usage instructions covers the typical concentrations, and addresses in detail a mixing phenomenon that can be observed during its preparation.

In my experience, each individual perceives the taste of a diluted, aqueous DMSO solution differently. People who want to take DMSO as a drink but find a preparation diluted only with water difficult to bear should try different fruit or vegetable juices to mask the taste. More on that in the section 'Oral administration'.

It is striking that DMSO's boiling and freezing points are much further apart than is the case with water. There is a difference of 170.5 °C between 189 °C and 18.5 °C. As we know, with water the difference is only 100 °C (which is astonishing for a substance with the low molar mass of 18 g/mol, and, as with DMSO, has to do with the fact that the

Fixed points water molecules are electrically polarised). As a result, DMSO assumes liquid form across a wide temperature range. This is associated with the so-called polarity of the individual DMSO molecules, which will be explained in more detail in the 'Chemical properties' section. Electrical polarity at the molecular level means that there is a strong pull between the liquid particles, making the transition to gas form by the addition of heat energy (= boiling point) more difficult. The relatively high boiling point of 189 °C that results is very practical because it prevents any loss of dimethyl sulfoxide to evaporation as you handle and use it at normal room temperatures. When you look at the overview table of physical properties above, this is conveyed by the very low vapour pressure at a temperature of 20 °C (compared with water). The section entitled 'External administration' explains why this fact is very helpful in terms of the application of DMSO via the skin.

DMSO's freezing point of around 18 °C often leads, to the amazement of (new) users, to supplies of the substance becoming solid overnight – particularly in winter when room temperatures fall. DMSO then looks like a block of ice inside the bottle, see (on the right) the figure below.

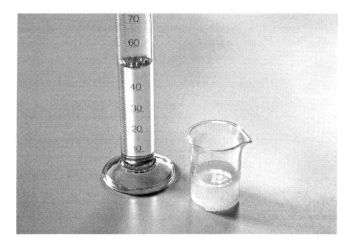

Figure 4: Liquid DMSO in a measuring cylinder; solid DMSO in a beaker

So do not be startled – a little time at a higher ambient temperature and the DMSO will return to a liquid state and be ready for use. There is no need to worry that the glass will shatter as the DMSO solidifies, as happens when water freezes, since DMSO does not expand in such a pronounced way as it freezes. Its expansion coefficient is only 0.0009. The figure for water is 0.21 (230 times higher), which is why water can cause bottles to shatter.

The density, or specific weight as it is still sometimes called, of DMSO is 10% higher than that of water. A litre of DMSO therefore weighs 1.1kg. This should be borne in mind in any quantity conversions for formulations, but it is otherwise not of any practical importance.

The weight of a certain number of DMSO molecules, namely Avogadro's constant, around $6 \cdot 10^{23}$ particles (= six with 23 zeroes behind it, so quite a big number), is more than four times that of water. This molar mass or molar weight (1 mol is equal to the quantity of $6 \cdot 10^{23}$ particles) is around 78 g/mol (= gram per mol). In addition to the strong pull that exists between particles that I mention above, the second reason why DMSO has a higher boiling point than water is because of the heavier mass of each individual DMSO molecule. As a point of comparison, the non-polar liquid hexane exhibits a much lower boiling point of only 69 °C despite having an even higher molecular mass of 86 g/mol.

DMSO's viscosity is double that of water. You can feel this clearly when *Viscosity* you rub a few drops of it between your fingers because we are so accustomed to the feel of water as a point comparison. Despite this, DMSO, and certainly all of its aqueous preparations, is still highly fluid. For some external applications, depending on what part of the body you are treating, this can be a disadvantage because the applied solution drips off too easily. We will discuss how this can best be resolved in the practical section of this book. Because of the low viscosity of DMSO the pharmaceutical industry has been very keen to develop gels and creams for external application. In my opinion that is not necessary because that is simply an indication that people do not want to wait the necessary time for the applied substance to be absorbed by the skin. But that is to forget that patience, care and attention are important elements in the treatment. This is just as true for self-treatment as it is for the interaction between doctor and patient.

The two parameters 'flash point' and 'ignition temperature' tell us that DMSO, in contrast to water, is an organic compound, and one that is flammable. You should therefore take care not to handle the liquid if there is an open flame nearby.

The possibility for acid dissociation, i.e. the readiness to separate a hydrogen atom from a methyl group of DMSO, is expressed by the pK_a value. This property is very weak in DMSO, which is why the value itself is higher than that of water (because it is a **negative**, decadic logarithm).

Carbon dioxide solution is a more common example of a compound that releases hydrogen ions – its pK_a value is correspondingly lower at 6.5. It is regarded as being a medium strength acid.

1.2.2 Chemical properties

Summary

DMSO 'gets on' with water just as well as it does with organic substances (fats, proteins, carbohydrates). This is an outstanding characteristic, the reasons for which lie in the liquid's molecular structure. Most other liquids **either** 'get along' better with water **or** with organic materials. You see this, for example, in the fact that water drips off a plastic surface (polyethylene) or that sugar (carbohydrate) is not soluble in olive oil.

Both inside and outside the cells of our bodies, and even on the boundary itself, we speak in terms of bio-organic structures made up of proteins, fats and carbohydrates (lipoproteins, proteoglycans, etc.) that are, for their part, dependent on an intact layer of water (hydration shell). It is because our body is, as a whole, a good mixture of water and organic substances that DMSO can achieve such a balancing and incisive effect. The chemistry of this substance shows us clearly why DMSO is able to have such a range of effects in the body. As a result, its healing power appears less as a coincidence and more as a natural piece of a puzzle, a happy stroke of fate …

As we approach the topic of the reactivity and the behaviour of DMSO towards organic tissue, it is helpful to examine the spatial structure of a

Molecular structure single molecule closely. Following the molecular formula depicted in section 1.1, one would tend to assume that DMSO is a planar particle, structured on a single level. In that case its ligands would be arranged on the paper plane around the central sulphur atom of this 'sulphur oxide compound'. In the case of the relevant 'carbon oxide compound', the highly toxic acetone, this really is true because carbon atoms, due to the structure of their electrons (fourth main group of chemical elements) can only establish a maximum of four atomic bonds.

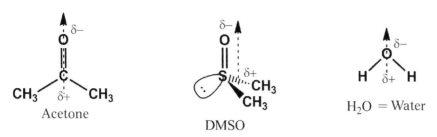

Figure 1 Dipolar substances in which the focus of the positive and negative partial charges do not match, even though they are electrically neutral towards the outside.

So in this case the double bond that is present, for which the central carbon atom and the oxygen atom each share two electrons, leads to a planar arrangement of the three groups of atoms. This ensures the greatest possible separation in this geometric, 'triangular' configuration.

In contrast, however, the central sulphur atom in dimethyl sulfoxide, as a member of the sixth main group of chemical elements, has the possibility of establishing up to six atomic bonds. This means that DMSO, where only four of the bonding possibilities have been used, still has two unused outer electrons. As a so-called free electron pair, these represent a fourth ligand. These are not usually taken into consideration in standard molecular diagrams (see figures 1 to 3). However, the presence of four neighbouring groups of atoms, positioned around a central sulphur atom inevitably leads (due to the reciprocal space requirements of these neighbours) to an arrangement that looks like the geometric figure of a pyramid. This is indicated in the figure above using the standard scientific symbols. Of course, it is not an exact, pyramid-shaped symmetry because the corners are formed by different ligands. The respective requirement for space is not only dependent on the purely calculative size of the neighbouring atoms / orbitals, but is also an expression of different electrostatic and quantum-mechanic effects. That is why the individual bond angles differ.

Furthermore, such interaction results in two different 'molecular edges', where the opposing charge densities on the atoms lead to the resulting total polarity of a DMSO molecule. While the position with the oxygen atom attracts negative charges to itself (O· high electronegativity), all that is left for the sulphur atom is to take on a positive partial charge (S· low electronegativity), or to partially transfer this electron attraction to

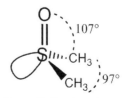

Figure 6: Bond angle

Polarity the methyl groups. Such a molecule is described therefore as being amphipathic overall, with a polar, hydrophilic ('water-loving') side and a predominantly nonpolar, hydrophobic terminal methyl group. The electron transfer between the oxygen atom and the rest of the molecule leads to the formation of what is known as a directional dipole moment, i.e. the formation of an axis with a positive (δ +) partial charge at one end and a negative (δ -) partial charge at the other, as shown in figure 5. So the whole molecule is an example of a bipolar particle, the DMSO as a liquid accordingly a bipolar solvent with a chain-like arrangement of the electrically aligned individual molecules. This 'ordering' of the liquid is also expressed in the dielectric permittivity of 49, for example, or in the very high electric dipole moment of 4.3 Debye (see table in section 1.2.1: water is 1.84 D). At the same time, this property determines the extraordinary solubilising power of other polar, ionic or at least polarisable substances.[17]

Structured liquids We have been familiar with the phenomenon of the inner structure of liquids for a long time, particularly with regard to water, our elixir of life (dielectric permittivity = 81), which is intensively researched with regard to this property both scientifically and parascientifically. Fortunately this effect is so pronounced in DMSO that it results in the high boiling point of 189 °C, as explained in the section on the substance's physical properties.

Water molecules in which the central oxygen atom has two bonding partners, namely two hydrogen atoms, do **not** therefore have a symmetrical, elongated structure.

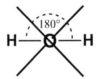

Figure 7: 'Wrong' H_2O molecule structure

Water would not otherwise cause an externally measurable dipole moment because such a symmetrical formation compensates for the effect of the partial charges. It is only due to the angular, triangular molecular structure (see figure 5, on the right) that the water molecule has a magnet-like behaviour with two opposing poles. This behaviour is very pronounced in both water and DMSO and leads, among other things, to a compatibility and communication between these two liquids in a biochemical sense.

Acetone, mentioned above, also displays a strong, observable polarity. This substance can also penetrate the skin easily (dipole moment of acetone: 2.9 D, so between DMSO and water). However, the most serious difference, in terms of its reactivity and behaviour in the body, is that acetone (which belongs to the ketone group) cannot oxidise further. The central carbon atom, as explained above, is saturated with bonds — no more oxygen atoms can be added. Acetone remains toxic because it is not affected by the body's detoxification processes and must be eliminated unaltered via the lungs and kidneys.

Furthermore, the sulphur atom, as a period three element, has higher energy orbitals at its disposal and is better able to balance the electron attraction of the oxygen atom than compounds such as acetone, in which a carbon atom forms the centre. It is, as we like to say, 'softer' and the aforementioned attraction of negative partial charges upon the two methyl groups is less sustained as a result. The result is that hydrogen atoms are significantly less likely to split off during chemical reactions (so-called acidity). It has a correspondingly high pK_a value of 35 in comparison with water's pK_a of 14, as listed in the table of physical properties (section 1.2.1).

Both the polarity and the low acidity make DMSO a highly valued, polar aprotic solvent. Aprotic means that it 'does not yield protons', whereby 'protons', in this case, stands for hydrogen ions more generally. *Excellent solvent* As a result, DMSO is regarded as a 'problem solver' when it comes to tricky dissolving challenges not only in medicine, where it is often mixed with various other substances to increase their effect, but also in research and industry. So unlike some of the alternative medicine scene's other highly effective treatments, dimethyl sulfoxide is not an insider secret. It is widely available in certified pharmaceutical quality, and doctors, vets and alternative practitioners can all vouch for the efficacy and safety of this substance.

Even if the exact reasons behind DMSO's extremely beneficial pharmacological properties are far from having been fully explained scientifically, they must somehow be connected to the spatial structure and the *Excellent carrier* special polarity at the molecular level. DMSO's superior ability to penetrate biological membranes and to transport other, dissolved substances with it as it does so, is also to be understood in this context. It has been discovered that positively charged substances (i.e. cations such as drug molecules, electrolytes, amino acids, etc.) dissolved in DMSO are surrounded by up to eight such bipolar particles.[18] A bigger assembly or aggregate forms as a result, which is characterised by an aligned shell, with the CH_3 groups of the DMSO molecule at the forefront. These CH_3 groups, however, are exactly those so-called organic parts of the sulf-oxide that likes to interact with other organic (i.e. containing hydrocar-bons) structures in biological tissue. DMSO's ability to displace individ-ual water molecules inside the body's cells can also be attributed to the molecule's special polarity. It means that the interaction between DMSO molecules and water molecules (H_2O), which are called hydro-gen bonds (see figure 10) are a little stronger than between two water molecules.

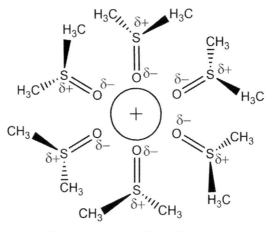

Figure 8: Cation with DMSO shell

The effect where particles are surrounded by polar, 'two-faced' sub-stances is generally called micelle formation and is just as common in cleaning agents as it is in our small intestines. In the case of the former, the dirt particles are surrounded by the surfactant molecules of the cleaning mixture and can then be easily washed out, i.e. be suspended in water. In the latter case, bile acid produced in the liver and the neutral fats from food form these spherical micelles so that the fats are more accessible to the digestive enzymes and can be absorbed more easily into the cells of the intestinal mucosa.

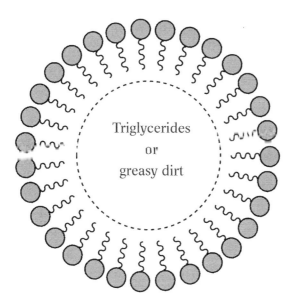

Figure 9: Micelle, e.g. from bile acid or surfactants

So it has hopefully become clear that it really is worth expanding your horizons to learn about the chemical properties of DMSO because this throws light on the fantastic versatility of the substance. Armed with this knowledge, you can proceed to the next chapter where we will finally be examining the tangible effects of this medicine. The pharmacological effects of this substance will then lead us directly and logically on to the areas of application, the diseases and conditions that can be treated using DMSO.

1.2.3 Pharmacological properties

Summary

The various effects of DMSO on humans and animals that have been discovered over many years of intensive research are extremely numerous. These effects can be divided into a few general categories: regeneration, penetration enhancer / carrier, protection and modulation. We really can speak here of a universal medicine. Some of the most significant effects include pain relief, the alleviation of inflammation, diuresis, vascular dilation, free radical scavenging, wound healing, and muscle relaxation. An important aspect of this is DMSO's ability to penetrate biological membranes such as the skin or cell walls with ease and to transport other (medicinal) substances with it as it does so.

In this context the term 'pharmacological' is taken to mean those properties that can be attributed to a substance retrospectively based on observable / measurable effects after it has been administered as a medication to humans or animals. In-vitro tests, i.e. tests carried out outside living organisms, for example on isolated tissue in laboratories, often deliver additional or independent results regarding the effects.

When referring to measurable effects, make certain that they are objectively ascertained and are statistically reproducible. There will of course be considerable individual variations, particularly when they are based on the personal appraisal of patients. One patient might describe the pain-relieving effect as being hardly discernible, another might claim a phenomenal, instant effect. Despite this, we should always strive to gather reliable treatment results.

Let us return to our example of the calcified shoulder joint. Looking beyond the joy the patient and the health practitioner feel when mobility is regained and the pain is relieved, the only truly acceptable way of judging the efficacy of DMSO treatment is by means of a positive result obtained from medical imaging methods. As alternative health practitioners we try to avoid resorting to diagnostic measures such as x-rays unless it is absolutely unavoidable. But we should remember that trumpeting allegedly swift cures achieved using complementary medicine can backfire when a subsequent conventional medical diagnosis provides a sobering wake-up call. Having said that, the subjective feelings of patients are given the highest priority – after all, they are seeking medical assistance because they want to feel better.

To put it plainly: the list of DMSO's tested and proven pharmacological properties is very long indeed. In fact, it is so long that it provokes critical responses from many. Some of these pharmacological properties may even appear to contradict one another. Even the fathers of the medical use of *Miracle* DMSO, which enjoyed such an impressive inception in the early 1960s, *medicine* now believe that the 'miracle medicine' label did more harm than good. But on closer inspection we see that many of the individual effects listed can be attributed to the same biochemical processes. Leaving to one side the use of DMSO as a supplement to other medicines for a moment, we can summarise the healing effects of DMSO, when used alone, as follows:

DMSO induces and supports the reorganisation and regeneration of cells, even in cases of severe damage to tissue, and protects the organism from developing a disease in the first place.

DMSO's 'comprehensive' healing effect is **unique** and may rightly be understood as an overarching treatment principle, as a singular and exceptional substance among medicines. There is no substitute for DMSO because of its vast range of properties that work harmonically together. Medical and pharmaceutical studies have repeatedly shown that DMSO has the largest number and the broadest range of effects ever proven for a single substance. Although we can choose between a number of substances that have the same or a similar effect in almost all other classes of substances, there is nothing that can replace DMSO.

Examining the list of effects attributable to DMSO that have so far been discovered is always a pleasure and it inspires us as we think of the application possibilities. I have compiled the list below using various sources and drawing from my practical experience. Dr Morton Walker's book *DMSO: Nature's Healer* (1993)[19] was particularly useful in this regard as it lists a number of indications / areas of application. Other useful sources include publications by Jacob and Herschler[20] and the overview article by Gerhards and Gibian.[8]

The following is a list of the pharmacological properties of DMSO that have been discovered so far – not in any particular order and with no claim to comprehensiveness.

- membrane-active, penetrates membranes in biological systems
- anti-inflammatory
- analgesic, nerve-blocking = pain-relieving
- bacteriostatic
- diuretic
- modulates and amplifies the effect of other drugs
- 'loosens up' connective tissue = anti-fibroplastic
- promotes diffusion of other substances = carrier, transportation function
- parasympathetic effect = suppresses acetylcholinesterase
- relaxant, promotes concentration
- vasodilatory = widens the blood vessels
- blocks calcium influx = increases myocardial contractility and ventricle function
- protects cells, e.g. from frost
- antioxidant = hydroxyl radical scavenger
- muscle relaxant
- improves cell function and cell differentiation
- anticoagulant, inhibits platelet aggregation
- modulates the blood lipids
- cell integration = protects in cases of blood circulation problems, radiation, hypothermia
- stabilises cell membrane e.g. from loss of plasma
- promotes wound healing
- heals scars, similar effect to collagenase = releases collagen
- anti-sclerotic
- improves breathing depth
- modulates the life cycle, division and apoptosis of cells
- changes permeability = influences the penetrability of tissue
- replaces water in cells
- improves oxygen saturation in tissue
- anti-anaemic effect

At this point, with readers probably stunned by DMSO's many healing properties, it should be reiterated that all these characteristics are attributable to the substance's molecular structure and the chemical and physical properties that were covered in the preceding sections. Even if it is often forgotten these days, on the sub-microscopic level we are still dealing – even in biological systems – with chemical reactions that proceed according to exact rules. Chemical reactions can be defined as changes in and interaction of individual molecules according to strictly specified formulae or chemical laws. This is still the case when we use the some-what more agreeable adjective 'biochemical'. Nature and life are and al-ways will be chemistry. This is the case with all the essential processes in plant (photosynthesis etc.) and animal cells. The liver, for example, is often appropriately described as the perfect chemical factory because of the way it converts or synthesises an almost unimaginable number of substances.

With regard to DMSO and its interactions in the tissue, we can hypoth- *Mode of* esise that the many healing effects listed above are attributable to the *action* molecule's ability to change the conformations, i.e. the spatial structures, of biomolecules and their hydration shells that it comes across. Current research attributes this primarily to the dipole characteristics outlined above and, more than anything, to the way it can form bonds with water and, even better, hydrogen.

From this we understand that DMSO molecules can replace individual water molecules in all biological hydrates, for example in protein struc-tures along with their hydration shells. An important example of this is cell membranes that, made up of up to 50% water, are highly ordered 'mixed structures' between lipoproteins and water. But because the newly attached DMSO molecules in such cell shells have a different

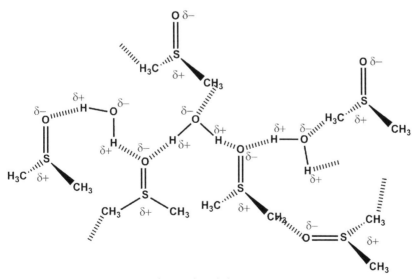

Figure 10: Hydrogen bonds between DMSO and H_2O

spatial structure and space requirement to the displaced water molecules, the conformation, i.e. the spatial arrangement, of the protein structures will also naturally change.

Because the main functions of these membrane structures, namely permeability for certain substances and the maintenance of an electrical potential, are dependent on their spatial arrangement, it is not at all surprising that DMSO is very efficient at modulating such processes. This is true for the analgesic effect, i.e. blocking pain stimuli along the peripheral nerves, for example. The sensitivity threshold of a nerve cell depends on its membrane potential and on the possibility for the swift migration of electrolyte ions (sodium Na^+, potassium K^+, etc.) from the inside out, or from the outside in.

Modulation

Because of the partial 'water replacement', other molecule or substance characteristics in the cell plasma or in the intracellular fluid change too, such as the osmotic effectiveness (= osmotic pressure) of electrolytes. This in turn influences the migration tendency of osmotically active particles with their hydration shells and can have a beneficial effect on the swelling in tissue inflammations because it increases the efflux of water.

Another possibility for DMSO to exert a modulating effect on protein structures in the body arises from the fact that, of the approximately 20 amino acids from which the body builds its protein structures, there are two that carry a sulphur atom. These are methionine and cysteine. The thiol groups contained within are, just like the hydration shells described above, responsible in large part for the spatial arrangement of proteins. The best known example is probably the chemical process required to 'perm' hair, whereby thiol groups in the hair proteins are changed. But the observable pharmacological properties of DMSO can also be partially understood in terms of the interaction with these sulphur-hydrogen-positions or even their chemical transformation.[21]

Based on what has so far been said, it can be inferred that, beyond the regenerative and balancing effect of DMSO, there must also be a toxic threshold because you cannot make an infinite number of changes to the body tissue. However, due to the conventional application methods used for human consumption, it is practically impossible to reach the toxic threshold as is sometimes done in animal or in-vitro experiments. Besides, the motto 'as little as necessary' should be your guiding principle, as with all alternative medicines.

As we try to gain a better understanding of DMSO's mode of action it will be helpful to remember that this liquid, due to its particular molecule characteristics, is always able to exchange places with water molecules.

Let us try a thought experiment: imagine that you are standing in the middle of a huge crowd of people and are allowed to exchange places with every second neighbour (our body is made up of at least 50% water, so every second molecule). It would be very easy for you to make your way through the crowd or to spend time at a certain spot talking to those around you if that is what you choose to do. Lingering in one spot and interacting in this way would result in other people turning around to face you, i.e. changing their spatial orientation. You could also take someone's hand and pull this person along behind you, taking every second position and 'flowing' comfortably through the crowd. As you move along in this way there is no grumbling and no one shouting 'don't push!' You are made welcome at the 'water spots' at all times and much attention is paid to you there. *Thought experiment*

DMSO molecules clearly come across very few barriers or resistance as they are distributed in the tissue / organs and they can linger at will, bringing about a relaxed feeling. These processes are only limited by the natural rate by which the body excretes the substance. All processes induced by DMSO are therefore reversible and by about the third day after application the substance is no longer present in the body.

To return to our image: once you have made your way through the crowd and are on your way home, all the spots are taken up by 'normal' people (water molecules) again and you no longer have an immediate effect on your neighbours.

However, some of them may well remember your presence there, or the modified spatial arrangements from before may now cause them to feel better as they stand there with their new neighbours. Figuratively speaking, DMSO has given the cell membrane a new or regained integrity. When we consider what would happen if a large number of such 'special' individuals advanced into a crowd of this kind (which represents biological tissue), enriching it, then it is easy to imagine how that would cause a regulating or loosening effect.

It is not known why the range of effects that DMSO has on body tissue is exclusively positive, or why other polar substances do not work in the same way, and are even poisonous in some cases. It is, ultimately, a peculiarity of nature, a coincidence (for the positivists among us) that we should accept with wonder and gratitude. *Coincidence*

Let us now return to the list of DMSO's numerous pharmacological properties. From this list of effects we can immediately identify the fields of application that were typically foregrounded during the early years of DMSO's therapeutic use and that continue to be important areas of use today. These include acute inflammatory diseases and trauma injuries such as sports injuries to the muscles, tendons and joints, inflammation in the joints, bursa and tendons, cervical brachial syndrome, or neuralgia, for example in connection with shingles (herpes zoster).[22]

The above explanation of the potential that DMSO displays on a molecular level helps us to understand the large number of (and the synergistic interaction between) different physiological effects the substance can have on these diseases. That is why I encouraged you in the introduction to read this chapter outlining the science behind the phenomena of DMSO.

Example of use   Let us take a concrete example of an acute sports injury to illustrate this point: a painful, dull trauma to the soft tissue (popularly called a 'Charley horse' in North America). When we treat this locally using a suitable DMSO solution, the first and most important effects are pain relief and reduction of swelling. However, DMSO's other properties are also important in terms of having a healing effect on this 'internal wound', not least the anti-inflammatory, vasodilatory, cell-protective, wound-healing, and muscle-relaxing effects. All these effects are attributable to DMSO's physical and chemical behaviour when faced with biological, hydrous cell systems. Accordingly, one should not analyse these individually, but rather consider their wonderfully regenerative effects as a synergistic whole.

Despite this, some of the individual pharmacological effects have been repeatedly subjected to studies in order to establish how they work and to prove their effectiveness. A number of the specially created animal models and study designs yielded reliable proof of the effects in question. Results of such studies have been presented at the 'Vienna DMSO Symposium of Scientists and Doctors' and published in countless scientific journals over the years. Some of this research will also be of interest to you because the studies have had a direct influence on the usage recommendations that have since been developed. One example of this is DMSO's diuretic effect, and another is its resorption and elimination behaviour (absorption and excretion rates).

The overview article by B. H. Ali (2001)[23] presents a summary of the scientific studies conducted on DMSO in the 1980s and the 1990s that were relevant to its basic pharmacological profile and therapeutic use. This expert declares that DMSO's singularly outstanding characteristic is its capacity to work as a free radical scavenger in damaged tissue, *Free radical* thereby reducing the oxidative stress that stands in the way of regener- *scavenger* ation. This kind of damage can occur in tissue following local distur- bances to the blood supply, as is often the case following strokes and coronary heart diseases.

Even if some authors sometimes foreground or emphasise a single mode of action, we should remember that these are only isolated ex- pressions of the general, astonishing capabilities of this substance, all of which arise from its molecular structure. This makes it possible for it to replace water molecules or to oxidise itself, thereby leading to a modulating reorientation on the molecular level throughout the whole organism.

Wood and Wood write in an article in 1975: 'Some of the studies to *DMSO puzzle* be reported in this monograph will describe additional, almost unbeliev- able observations. Perhaps the mechanism of action of these clinical phenomena will be found in one or more of the pharmacological prop- erties described. It would not be surprising, however, if we were to con- clude with a resolution to search for new explanations of the mystery of DMSO, for it would appear that DMSO is really a new principle in med- icine and cannot always be measured by existing standards.'[24] In this article, Wood and Wood specifically emphasise the significance of DMSO's ability to penetrate membranes.

Let us take a closer look at the most important of DMSO's medicinal effects.

DMSO's **antioxidant** properties derive primarily from its ability to 'deactivate' hydroxyl radicals (OH·) through chemical reaction. The DMS (see section 1.1) that is formed in the human body in small quan- tities can also trap oxygen radicals (O·).[20] These damage the tissue and *Antioxidation?* are produced in cases of ischemia (circulatory / oxygen insufficiency), inflammations, traumas, etc. The mechanisms by which hydroxyl radi- cals are captured have recently been the subject of impressive studies by Baptista et al.[25] and other researchers.[26]

We can therefore assume (to state in simplified terms) that OH radicals and DMSO first form a complex that is stabilised by water molecules.

A methyl radical ($CH_3\cdot$) and sulphinic acid (CH_3SOOH) then usually emerge from this complex. The methyl radical has various possibilities in terms of further reactions. It can either bond with its own kind to become ethane, or it can steal a hydrogen atom from another DMSO molecule to form methane, or it can form a peroxide with oxygen.

In all these cases the exact reaction processes depend heavily on the particular conditions in the body tissue (pH level, oxygen supply, water saturation, etc.). What is crucially important is the fact that DMSO 'picks up' radical metabolic products and neutralises their ability to harm. The body can eliminate the compounds that are subsequently formed via the excretion pathways. The positive effects that result are also ascribed to DMSO's anti-inflammatory and pain-relieving characteristics. It also appears that oxygen supply to the cells improves as a result.

Inflammation inhibition DMSO's **anti-inflammatory** effect (primarily on acute injuries) is evidently largely due to its inhibitory and synthesis-blocking properties against inflammation mediators (prostaglandin, interleukin, etc.); it therefore induces a balancing or restricting effect on cell-mediated immune defence processes. The movement of inflammation cells is also apparently inhibited.[27, 28]

The **immune-modulating** effect can be attributed to the same cause. If we recall the five tell-tale signs of inflammation from the pathology textbooks, it becomes clear why the anti-inflammatory properties of DMSO are so effective when treating acute conditions. These five signs are: swelling, redness, hyperthermia, pain and functional impairment. These local symptoms and developments in the affected tissue are caused, generally speaking, by the inflammation mediators and inflammation cells mentioned above. Having said that, the general inflammation process is useful as a physiological ('normal') reaction by the body when faced with a pathological (disease-causing) stimulus. The (warning) pain and the functional impairment following an acute injury naturally serve to remind us to rest and protect the affected area.

Nevertheless, complete healing can only occur when inflammation processes have ceased. That is why DMSO can be useful in the treatment of the following conditions: swellings and pains after acute injuries to the musculoskeletal system; *Diseases of the central nervous system* acute / traumatic diseases of the central nervous system (brain and spinal cord); diseases caused by microorganisms (septic) and rheumatic diseases, as well as other autoimmune diseases of the connective tissue.

However, it should be borne in mind, particularly with regard to sports injuries, that if the patient is free of pain and function is restored quickly, the bones and the muscles may not be able to manage being subjected to strain once again so soon. It is important in such cases to consult an experienced sports therapist. Where professional sport is involved there is a danger that the health of the individual, be it a person or an animal (e.g. performance horses), is sacrificed for financial reasons. As a health practitioner or a self-user you should not capitalize on living beings.

It has been established in experiments that the **pain-relieving** (analgesic) *Pain relief* effect of DMSO can be attributed to the way it reduces the neural impulse pathways, i.e. slows nerve conduction velocity or even blocks what is known as the C fibres.[29] These are the 'slow', pain-sensing nerve fibres that have a conduction velocity of 0.5 to 2.0 metres per second. This is not an anaesthetic in the conventional sense since a needle prick in the affected tissue will still be felt. DMSO is therefore not an anaesthetic and neurological tests remain positive.

A number of authors emphasise that the pain-relieving effect is also attributable to DMSO's ability to catch free radicals and / or its anti-inflammatory effect because these stop the actual processes that cause the pain.[9] Jacob and Rosenbaum observed that the pain relief usually sets in 30 to 60 minutes after DMSO is administered and remains effective for 4 to 6 hours; the pain is usually less intense once it returns (modulation / regeneration).

The **membrane-active** or **membrane-penetrating** properties of DMSO derive from the substance's ability to easily penetrate biological barriers such as skin, cell walls, cell organelle membranes, bacterial walls and the blood–brain barrier.[30] The previous section explained how this is *Frontier* mainly attributable to the amphipathic character of the DMSO mole- *crosser* cule, which is a result of its polarity and the presence of both methyl groups. Think back to the image in our thought experiment when you made your way through a crowd of people by exchanging places with others.

However, DMSO has an additional distinctive feature. As it makes its way through biological membranes it can take other substances, such as the molecules of other medicinal substances, with it. Its ability to do so depends on the size, form and charge of the particular medicine.

43

DMSO is therefore very useful as a solvent and carrier of other active agents.[9]

In fact, in the few commercial medicinal preparations available today that contain DMSO, this is practically the only effect that is intentionally taken advantage of – for example, increasing the absorption / penetration and efficacy of cortisone (glucocorticoids), e.g. Dexamethason in DMSO®, CP-Pharma. The effect of cortisone can be increased by between 10 and 1000 times in this way. Very small quantities of DMSO would suffice for this 'taxi function', quantities that would, unaided, be too low to bring about DMSO's own intrinsic medicinal effects.

In alternative medicine, DMSO is also used as a transporter when MMS is applied externally. Read more about this approach in Dr Antje Oswald's *The MMS Handbook: Your Health in Your Hands*. MMS is a liquid solution that has a selective oxidative effect and which is used to treat infectious diseases and cancer.

We can also use DMSO's function as a carrier of predominantly low-molecular substances to treat damage to tissue. To do so, dissolve procaine in DMSO; this mixture can be used to treat scars without using needles, which has at least two major benefits (more on this in the practical section).

Caution   At this point we should add a note of warning with regard to DMSO's ability to transport other substances as it moves in and through the skin. Textile dyes, for example, can cause serious skin irritation, or even more harmful symptoms. This issue is covered in detail in the practical section of this book.

Other characteristics   As was the case regarding DMSO's analgesic effect, a number of different specific mechanisms lie behind its **anti-ischemic** effect (i.e. protection from circulation and oxygen deficiencies). These mechanisms include anticoagulation (**antithrombotic** because it inhibits platelet aggregation),[31,32] expansion of blood vessels (**vasodilatory**),[33] protection of the inner lining of the blood vessels (vascular endothelial function) through suppression of deposits and agglutination (adhesions),[34] and improved oxygen diffusion.[35] The **diuretic** effect of DMSO[36,37] also contributes to promoting perfusion and circulation in damaged organs as soon as the tissue fluid pressure reduces as the swelling subsides.

The best protection against damage resulting from insufficient perfusion is to provide the tissue with DMSO in advance.[10] This appears to be sound advice, but raises the question of whether it is possible to foresee an impending stroke. That is certainly not so in all cases, but a patient's case history can often provide important signs that indicate elevated risk of illness resulting from an undersupply of oxygen / nutrients to the affected tissue, and poor elimination of metabolic waste products. This is just as true for the typical arteriosclerotic diseases (coronary heart disease / heart attack, peripheral arterial occlusive disease, etc.) as it is for intestinal colic, in which case DMSO remedies insufficient supply to the intestinal walls.[38] All this is quite apart from the fact that DMSO has anti-sclerotic effects of its own.[39]

DMSO can modulate the activity of some of the enzymes produced naturally in the body. This can be understood in terms of DMSO's ability, explained above, to change the spatial molecular configuration of protein structures and / or their hydration shells. The enzymes' ability to drastically accelerate biochemical reactions is due to the perfectly 'fitting' spatial formation of the reaction centre. Both reaction partners in the chemical transformation must reach this centre and find one another so that an optimum interaction can occur. *Enzyme effect*

Think of it as a half-open cavity that is formed when you bring your fingertips together and press down into dough. Even minor spatial changes to a 'molecule hollow' of this kind changes the properties of an enzyme. This change is particularly dramatic in relation to the specific acceleration rate of the respective metabolic reactions. DMSO's **para-sympathetic** effect is derived from this characteristic.

What does all this mean? It is quite simple. Our autonomic or involuntary nervous system normally controls the functions of the organs without our conscious awareness. The autonomic nervous system is comprised of two parts: the sympathetic and the parasympathetic nervous systems. When we are in an ergotropic phase, i.e. when we are required to take action, the influence of the sympathetic part of the autonomic nervous system predominates. This leads, for example, to increases in heart rate and breathing, expansion of the bronchia, the coronary blood vessels and the pupils, and causes the peripheral blood vessels to contract, causing blood pressure to rise. Many books describe this as the 'fight-or-flight response', as discovered by the American physiologist and stress researcher Walter Cannon. This is the evolutionary response that allowed us to survive dangerous encounters with sabre-toothed cats in the distant past.

After a successful prehistoric mammoth hunt, when the work is done and the feast prepared, the parasympathetic part of the autonomic nervous system comes into play. This part supports the work of the digestive glands and the intestinal peristaltic, while slowing down the heart and breathing rate. This is the trophotropic phase, which is generally directed towards nourishment, digestion and regeneration.

Relaxation   When we say that DMSO has a parasympathetic effect, this means that it increases the activity of the parasympathetic nervous system. In other words, DMSO has a calming effect because it guides the interplay between the two parts of the autonomic nervous system towards the parasympathetic side. This parasympathetic side, as explained above, is the side responsible for the resting and regeneration phases of the body and its organs, i.e. for the stress-free periods in the physiological sense.

How does DMSO do this? It inhibits the exact enzyme that is responsible for hydrolysing the parasympathetic neurotransmitter acetylcholine into its inactive form.[40] DMSO changes the acetylcholinesterase spatially to such an extent that its activity (i.e. its ability to increase the rapidity with which the anti-stress signals in the tissue are overcome) is significantly reduced. The sympathetic nervous system's influence, as the stress catalyst of the autonomic system, is thus diminished because it makes use of another neurotransmitter, namely noradrenalin, for its effect on the effector organs.

Considering the average person's lifestyle in this modern age, it is instantly clear that a medical substance that has a calming, stress-reducing effect and a whole host of other positive properties could be extremely useful. But moving beyond this admittedly simplistic conclusion, the parasympathetic metabolic state (i.e. a phase of regeneration and nourishment) is vitally important for beginning the healing process following an acute illness or injury.

Its **enzymatic effects** are perhaps the most interesting aspects of this substance. Other examples of such effects include the inhibition of alcohol dehydrogenase[41] and the support of the activity of the enzyme collagenase.[42] In the case of the former, the effect of DMSO practically increases the effect of the (potable-) alcohol (ethanol) because the liver enzyme that is responsible for the detoxification reaction of this substance is inhibited. That does not sound particularly advantageous. However, alcohol dehydrogenase also plays an important role in a number of other breakdown processes in the liver, meaning that its impact has even more important consequences than the intoxication effect.

In contrast, DMSO's promotion of collagenase activity has more *DMSO and* obviously advantageous effects. As its name suggests, collagenase plays *the connective* an important role as a degrading enzyme of collagen-rich connective *tissue* tissue structures. Collagen is the most abundant protein in our bodies and it is a key component of all connective tissue such as tendons, ligaments, bones, cartilage, teeth and skin. It forms their extracellular matrix, the 'jointing mortar' or 'scaffold structure', so to speak. The function cells and the matrix are permanently exchanging signals and substances, the significance of which has only recently been properly established. This substance within the intercellular space is produced by specialist cells, such as fibre forming cells (fibroblasts) or bone forming cells (osteoblasts).

It is important that a constant balance is established between the controlled formation and decomposition of such connective tissue. Taking bones as an example, the whole structure is constantly regenerated / rebuilt or adjusted to changing conditions by means of the interplay between the osteoblasts and the osteoclasts (cells that resorb bone tissue).

You may have heard that astronauts returning from space suffer from softening of the bones after spending long periods at zero gravity because the bone structure is not exposed to the same demands as those made upon it on Earth. When the astronauts return to Earth the specialist cells start work to adapt the bone structure to the new conditions.

When these processes occur in the body, it is vital that the collagen is not produced in excessive amounts. That is why we need collagenase. If the synthesis and breakdown of this stabilising tissue is out of balance, it leads to pathological processes. Some examples include:

- hypertrophic scars, i.e. scars that thicken and become raised
- keloid formation, i.e. scars that expand beyond the injured area
- formation of adhesions, i.e. scar tissue in the abdominal cavity that form following injury during surgery (danger of intestinal lumen obstruction)
- excessive callus formation following bone fractures, potentially causing wound contracture (constriction and functional limitation).

It is clear that DMSO is an extremely useful substance when it comes to improving scar tissue. It strides effortlessly across the borders between the blood vessels, function cells and the matrix, and as a result it exerts a corresponding level of influence on the formation of (new) connective tissue. Old scars can be minimized and softened, and their appearance reduced effectively using DMSO.

Personally, however, I believe that the treatment of internal scars is a far more important issue than the cosmetic aspect. DMSO can be used to accelerate healing and regeneration following accidents, injuries and (abdominal) operations. The risk of post-operative adhesion formation is reduced. The scar tissue (both internally and externally) becomes qualitatively improved and more flexible / supple. It is not only the collagenase-like effect that is decisive here. The inhibition of the above-mentioned fibroblasts, and the reduced formation of inferior granulation tissue in which collagen accumulates, are also conducive to the improved healing of wounds and injuries.[39]

We can speculate that some of the other properties of DMSO listed above also have a positive effect in this regard. These would include the anti-inflammatory, circulation stimulating, and antioxidant effects. After all, the cross-linking reaction in which individual collagen molecules transform into mechanically resilient fibrils includes an oxidative step.

Improved oxygen supply

Improved oxygen saturation in the tissue is presumably the result of a number of synergistic DMSO properties.[19,43] James Finney's extremely interesting study includes a description of how an infusion solution of DMSO and hydrogen peroxide (H_2O_2) sustains the functionality of the heart musculature in tests on narcotized pigs and rabbits, even though the coronary blood supply was inhibited. It appears that no one followed up on this astonishing experimental approach at the time. Hydrogen peroxide, like DMSO, is not lucrative and its medicinal use has been almost completely ignored for a long time. However, DMSO's oxygen saturation effect, together with the effect of promoting diffusion, is presumably based on some of its other properties. These could be the expansion of local blood vessels and capillaries, and reduced platelet aggregation (i.e. improved blood flow). Both are prerequisites for an optimised supply of oxygen and nutrients to the cells.[44]

The **bacteriostatic, antiviral and antifungal** effects of DMSO have been tested on a number of very different microorganisms. Between 30 and 40% aqueous solutions have been shown to effectively inhibit the growth of Pseudomonas, *Staphylococcus aureus* and Escherichia coli.[16] A number of other laboratory tests prove that diluted DMSO solutions, by themselves, fight bacteria, viruses and fungi. Furthermore, DMSO improves the distribution of other antimicrobial substances, thereby enhancing their potential effect.

Without needing to go deeper into these physiological processes, it is already clear that DMSO should not be regarded as a simple medicinal product, but that it possesses a wealth of complex modulating properties. What at first appear to be conflicting effects actually complement each other, offering a balancing, therapeutic approach for the treatment of a number of physical processes that have fallen out of balance.

1.2.4 Safety of the medicinal product

Summary

DMSO is regarded as a very safe and well-tolerated medication. Countless clinical and experimental trials have been carried out, a large number of which were conducted decades ago. DMSO has been tested and implemented as a medicinal treatment since the 1960s and the number of people treated with the substance is enormous.

There are no true adverse effects except for DMSO's 'special' side effect, namely the odour (caused by a decomposition product) that can be detected for about 1½ days after it is taken. When DMSO is used externally as a diluted solution it can cause temporary redness and flaking of the skin or itching because of its vasodilatory effect. This effect varies from person to person and depends on the area of the body treated. It is usually more pronounced in people who have pale skin and less pigmented irises. Weaker dilutions can be used to balance this, or the skin can be soothed after application using water or skincare products.

The LD50 value of DMSO – an (inverse) measure of a substance's poisonousness that is arrived at using animal experiments – shows that it is far safer than ibuprofen, aspirin, caffeine and even cooking salt. Nevertheless, one should remain cautious and always carry out a tolerance test before using the substance for the first time or test out the DMSO for each user.

'DMSO is seven times safer than aspirin' – that was the conclusion of a study comparing the data from various medical experiments.[19] Why the comparison with aspirin (or acetylsalicylic acid / ASA)? Firstly, it is a reference point that almost everyone will be familiar with because it is a drug that can be bought easily everywhere. The second reason why aspirin is a particularly appropriate comparison is that DMSO, in the early days, was introduced and prescribed mainly for pain relief and as an anti-inflammatory medicine, as a peroral and intravenous alternative to aspirin.

America's painkiller   During the 1960s word spread so quickly concerning this that many people in North America continued to take DMSO on their own responsibility even during the temporary period when DMSO prescription was halted due to the incorrect interpretation of the animal studies mentioned in the introduction. After treating rabbits, pigs and dogs using what were in some cases excessive quantities of DMSO, some of the animals became short-sighted. This effect has never been replicated in higher mammals or humans, or when used at normal dosages.

Tens of thousands of people continued to buy DMSO, some of them acquiring poor DMSO from dubious sources and at inflated prices. Although we can assume that many took the cheap, so-called 'technical grade' DMSO, there are no reports of serious incidents from this period.

This story is reminiscent of the unsuccessful period of Prohibition in the USA between 1919 to 1932, when the ban on alcohol led to a booming black market. The poor quality of the illegal drink (containing high levels of methanol and fusel oils) certainly damaged people's health – quite apart from the fact that alcohol (ethanol) is not a medicinal substance and is toxic even in low doses. It is clear that the authorities had not learnt the lessons of the Prohibition period; they thought they could deprive the population of this new painkiller by means of official regulations.

Dr Morton Walker writes in his book *DMSO: Nature's Healer* (1993): 'The drug has been in public use underground since 1964, employed by tens of thousands of Americans, and up to now no toxicity has been reported in consumer reports, at medical meetings, in the scientific literature, during the four international DMSO symposia, or anywhere else. The approximately 2,000 people for whom physicians in medical practice have personally prescribed DMSO have not advised of any serious deleterious reactions. Yes, there are minor side effects, which I will discuss, that are outweighed by the many DMSO benefits. But toxicity or ill health arising from its use? None at all!' (p. 74).[19]

Medications and, by now, many other substances must undergo extensive toxicity tests (European REACH legislation). In DMSO's case these were carried out on fish, birds and mammals (including humans).[45] To summarise the results, we can say that it is difficult to es- *Safety* tablish what the toxic threshold is because it is usually impossible to obtain the necessary quantity of DMSO that would trigger ascertainable damage to health into an organism in the first place. For example, rats were submersed in a 60% solution three times a week for 26 weeks and remained totally healthy.[46] The established toxicity of a substance is defined by what is known as its LD_{50} value. This figure indicates what quantity of the substance is required (in milligrams per kg of body weight) to cause half (50%) of all the test subjects (e.g. small fish) to die.

Note: The higher a substance's LD_{50} value, the safer it is!

Because it is practically impossible to arrive at a meaningful result for DMSO use on laboratory animals whose physiology is roughly comparable to that of humans, LD_{50} values were often based on estimates. As a result they have, in my opinion, very little significance, except for the message that what we have here is an extremely safe substance. For example, the LD_{50} value of DMSO when administered orally (by drinking) to dogs is estimated to be higher than 10,000(!). That means that a dog weighing 20kg would have to drink 200 grams of pure DMSO to create a high probability of triggering any kind of harmful effect. That is more than 180 millilitres! It is hard to imagine that any dog would drink that kind of quantity.

Although the meaningfulness of such studies can certainly be questioned in terms of their applicability to humans, they suggest that a person weighing 70kg would need a dose of 700g of DMSO. This is, of course, utter nonsense! Even the corresponding figure for monkeys, which is estimated at above 4,000, would still mean a dose of 280 grams for the average human before they had a 50% risk of experiencing severe toxicity. If you consumed such quantities of salt, tea or sugar, no one would be surprised if you experienced toxic reactions or metabolic imbalances. The table below lists the LD_{50} values taken from comparable experiments on rats, figures that are often used on safety instruction leaflets:

Cooking salt:	3,000mg/kg
Calcium hypochlorite (MMS 2):	850mg/kg
Ibuprofen (Nurofen® etc.):	636mg/kg
Chlorine dioxide (MMS / CD):	292mg/kg
ASA (Aspirin® etc.):	200mg/kg
Caffeine:	192mg/kg
Nicotine:	50mg/kg
But: MSO:	14,500mg/kg!

When you consider how casually and excessively painkillers such as ibuprofen are used by adults and even by children these days, you will probably smile when you come across the 'safety instructions' assiduously distributed by the authorities and industry with regard to the self-administration of DMSO as a medicinal product (or MMS, which is safer than acetylsalicylic acid and caffeine). The fact is that anyone who searches for unbiased information and takes responsibility for their own health (and / or seeks advice from a holistic healthcare practitioner) is not going to be a lucrative customer / patient for the pharmaceutical industry. With DMSO costing about 25 pence per day of treatment and with patients buying it directly, the pharma industry is going to miss out.

Low treatment costs Having said that, the pharma giants themselves pounced on DMSO in the 1960s. If only it did not cause that smell … The predicted profits were also deemed to be too low when compared with the expense involved in producing the required data for the official approval procedure.[*]

Today, DMSO is enjoying a comeback, having been rediscovered by the field of alternative medicine. For a long time it was only used by doctors working in specialist fields or who only treated private patients. It is understandable that some will be irritated by DMSO's belated success, thinking of all the missed opportunities. Say what you will about the smell – you have to decide for yourself what does you good and what is most important to you!

In this respect the history of DMSO reminds me a little of the pharmacists who, during the early days of motoring, were given an opportunity to sell petrol alongside their traditional business. After trying it out and deeming it to be too much hassle or not befitting their status, they stopped selling it – perhaps also due to the smell. They simply lacked the imagination to foresee how developments in motoring would change

---

[*] News: As of November 2015 DMSO ampules are officially available in Germany!

our world, all because the number of people who could afford an 'automobile' was small initially and their numbers increased only very slowly. They were impatient and lacked vision.

Other toxicity studies have shown that DMSO does not cause cancer,[47] is not a teratogen,[48] and is not an allergen.[49]

It is far more productive to examine those experience reports and study results where therapeutically reasonable quantities of DMSO have been used on humans, for example, the study by R. D. Brobyn,[50,51] who carried out a high-profile application experiment in 1967–68 on more than 100 healthy prisoners aged between 21 and 55 in California. They were (only) given a dose that is about 3 to 30 times higher than the standard daily dose today, and that over a period of 14 or 90 days. The first group was given a daily dose of 1g per kg of body weight (1000mg/kg) *90-day trial* in the form of an 80% gel via the skin. This quantity and concentration was still very high and 13 of the 78 volunteers who initially started the trial had to be excluded after the first two applications due to excessively severe skin irritation.

The remarkable thing is that the other 65 test subjects were able to tolerate so much DMSO on the skin. One participant who weighed 80kg was given a daily dose of 80 grams. None of the tests (blood counts, neurological tests, heart-circulation parameters and eye examinations) carried out before, during or after treatment indicated any kind of toxic effect.

In the second group, 54 subjects were given an equally high daily dose of DMSO, in this case for a period of three months. Twelve of the test persons in this group had to be excluded from the study because their skin was too sensitive to the high-concentration gel. A further two dropped out due to the odour and for personal reasons. In total, 40 people were given 1000mg/kg of DMSO for 90 days. All the physical tests carried out on this group, which were more extensive than the tests carried out on the 14-day group, confirmed that DMSO should be classed as a safe substance. After all, the 90-day test subjects had been given, on average, a total of 8kg of pure DMSO over this period. Would we be able to tolerate other common household substances and medications in these quantities?

There was a small number of slight changes, randomly distributed across the control group, in individual blood parameters, as well as temporary bouts of headache and tiredness. However, these did not stop anyone from continuing with the trial. Following the trial, Brobyn and his colleagues were in no doubt that they had confuted the questionable 'eye degeneration' myth once and for all, proving that DMSO's useful effects far outweighed the side effects that had at times been observed. As you will read in the practical section of the book, the usage recommendations we adhere to today are actually based on lower, effective total quantities, and individual concentrations of the preparations. Despite that, you should consider seeking the advice of an experienced practitioner, particularly when suffering from a serious illness or when using DMSO internally or over long periods of time.

You should also be aware that there is no promise of a cure where DMSO use is concerned – no treatment can promise success. There are numerous cases of so-called 'non-responders', patients who do not respond to a treatment in the desired or expected way. It is relatively easy to test DMSO on your own responsibility because all the observations made so far confirm that it is well tolerated and the success rate, compared with some standard treatments, is very high. The chances of an improvement in your health are high and we have a number of reports of cures.

As an alternative health practitioner I can only justifiably recommend a substance and write a book about it if I have personally had excellent results using it. After all, our profession is governed by a set of ethical guidelines. That is true both for self-treatment and when administering the substance to family members, friends, acquaintances and patients. *Self-treatment* Because we are discussing a patent-free substance that is widely available at affordable prices, it should be clear that there is no business interest behind my recommendation, as we sadly often suspect is the case with many conventional medicines and their many side effects. Fortunately, this issue is discussed publically these days. Whether that is enough to hold the rampant 'health industry' in check and to protect patients remains doubtful.

Now that you have some knowledge of DMSO as a potent but well tolerated medicine that has a wide range of pharmacological effects, it is up to you to consider whether to use it on yourself or your patients. You can use it both as a single medication or mixed with other substances to intensify their effect. When doing so, always bear in mind your responsibility towards yourself and others. In cases of severe illnesses, seek the advice of experts who work holistically when possible. The practical aspects of how exactly to use this 'liquid healer', and the necessary requirements for doing so, are discussed in the following chapter.

Therapeutic Application

Countless scientific articles from across the globe confirm that DMSO is a very safe substance that can be used to treat a wide range of conditions. Both the treatment results described in the scientific literature, and my own experiences and the experiences of colleagues in the health professions, indicate that DMSO often quickly succeeds in bringing about an amazing initial improvement in the context of a range of diseases and symptoms. Unfortunately this leads some people to place all their hopes of a cure on DMSO. However, as is generally understood in the world of holistic alternative medicine, such initial results are often followed only by limited progress if the patient fails to work on the cause of imbalance on all levels – body, mind and spirit.

A sudden reduction in symptoms, or even their complete disappearance, does not absolve you of the duty you have to your physical body and the consciousness that resides within it. Dietary and life habits must be examined and reviewed, as should your thinking habits. The exact *Think* scope of the psychogenic influence of the mind on long-term disease *holistically* processes is still not fully understood. The cerebrum of the *Homo sapiens* may have accomplished a host of technical and cultural wonders ('… and they ate from the tree of knowledge …') and it has, according to Darwin, given us an important evolutionary advantage. However, the other side of the coin is often forgotten, namely that the cerebrum is at the same time a great burden for us because thoughts, as neuronal processes in the cerebral cortex, alongside the hormones, (can) significantly restrict our supposed freedom of action.

Just as the road to illness can be very short (accidents) or very long (chronic, stealthy processes), there is a road back to health. Sudden and immediate cures are, understandably, in great demand but they cannot be guaranteed!

The road leading out of a (physical) crisis, as you probably know from personal experience, often involves personal development. You can therefore use DMSO as a precursor, a boost to the body's own regeneration processes. However, you should think in holistic terms when treating yourself or others so that you can achieve a genuine, permanent cure. It should be clear to everyone that a case of shoulder–arm syndrome that developed as a result of excessive stress on one side while working over many years will return if the same problematic activity is repeated (too soon) after being successfully treated with DMSO. Likewise, it cannot be expected that patients suffering from states of exhaustion (burnout / bore-out), fibromyalgia or chronic bowel diseases will ever be completely rid of their symptoms if, following an initial improvement, they forget to treat the emotional element of their illness.

2.1 GENERAL INSTRUCTIONS OF USE

Before going into the practical details of how to use DMSO, a few general tips will be given here. DMSO is not available in pharmacies as an individual medication approved for human use. In Germany, DMSO is only available in a mixture with heparin and dexpanthenol in the form of a gel for external use (Dolobene Gel® / Merckle Recordati). The quantity of DMSO contained in this product is rather low and is mainly intended to improve the tissue penetration rate of the other two substances.

Regarding veterinary products the situation is quite different. There are at least four products on the market, all of them combinations of DMSO and other substances, and intended for external application on pets. Dexamethason in DMSO®, a treatment for inflamed joints and produced by the CP-Pharma company, is very popular with veterinarians. This contains 990mg of DMSO per millilitre, indicating a certain confidence in DMSO's effectiveness as a medicine in its own right. The other products are Phlogamed® (Alma Pharma), Prurivet - S® (Vétoquinol) and Otiprin N®(Vétoquinol); these are drops to treat ear infection in dogs.

Buying DMSO If you wish to use DMSO as an individual substance (without cortisone etc.) on humans or animals, or if you wish to prepare your own combinations of DMSO with other substances, you should buy pure DMSO from one of the many internet retailers that sell it. You can usually buy it in quantities of 100ml to 1 litre, which you will certainly need in order to carry out your first experiments with DMSO. When stored away from light and at a temperature of below 20 °C, pure DMSO keeps for a long time. You can tell that a substance is of pharmaceutical quality from the letters 'Ph. Eur.', an abbreviation of 'European Pharmacopoeia'. Compliance to these standards is monitored by the European Pharmacopoeia Commission. You can obtain quantities larger than 1 litre from chemical suppliers, but that probably only makes sense if you are working as a health practitioner or are treating large animals. Prices demanded by the various internet retailers are quite similar and there is very little difference in quality between solutions of 99.7% and above.

It would be unwise to publish here a list of outlets where you can buy DMSO – that would be to saw off the branch one is sitting on. As the example regarding MMS has shown, retailers come under immense pressure when people imprudently and vociferously announce in books or on internet forums that certain substances can be bought in particular places. The case of MMS is somewhat different because the basic substance used to prepare the solution is officially classed as a dangerous substance and its sale to private customers is therefore subject to certain regulations.

Despite that, the alternative medicine community does itself no favours when it unnecessarily draws the attention of the 'higher powers' to reliable suppliers. I will leave the question of who is behind the repercussions (that include website warning letters, search term repression, company audits, etc.) to your imagination. DMSO is in any case completely safe, the bottles do not carry safety warnings, and there are no restrictions on sales to private customers.

Once you obtain your first bottle of DMSO, take care from the very beginning to keep everything scrupulously clean so as not to contaminate the content. It is best to draw small quantities from the container using a clean, graduated pipette. Laboratory suppliers sell Pasteur *Cleanliness* pipettes for this purpose; these are (single-use) pipettes made of plastic, with millilitre markings on the stem. You can, of course, use these more than once as long as you keep them clean. Reusable glass pipettes in various sizes are a possible alternative. If using these you will also need a Peleus ball made of rubber in order to draw up the required quantity of DMSO before emptying it into another container. These graduated glass pipettes are longer than the plastic pipettes, which means that you can usually draw the DMSO up from the very bottom of the bottle. In contrast, when using a short pipette you often have to hold the bottle at an angle when it is almost empty in order to reach the remaining liquid.

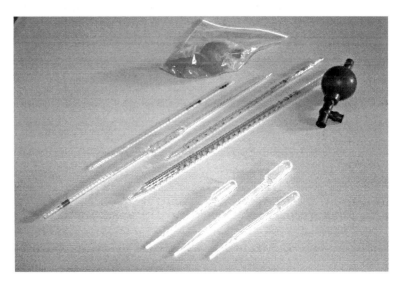

Figure 11: Various measuring pipettes

Note: Pure DMSO – **undiluted** – is a vaporous, flammable liquid that can cause irritation to the mucous membranes. It can also cause eye irritation. When undiluted it must always be stored in closed containers and kept out of the reach of children. It should also be stored away from sources of ignition, hot surfaces and flames. You should not inhale the vapour or spray mist. If the substance gets into the eyes, rinse thoroughly for a few minutes under flowing water and with the eyes open. You should wear protective glasses when pouring pure DMSO. If swallowed accidentally, you should rinse out the mouth and drink plenty of water to prevent irritation of the mouth, throat or the oesophagus membranes. The dilutions of DMSO with water suggested in the following chapter should be easily tolerated by the respective areas of the body. If the area treated becomes irritated, you can quickly alleviate the symptoms by adding water at any time.

When using larger containers such as those seen in medical centres, it is advisable to purchase a dispenser made from a suitable material from a laboratory supplier. This is a type of piston pump which you can configure to extract a preset quantity when you press the pump.

Such a dispenser is relatively expensive so I will suggest an alternative method of extracting DMSO (or other liquids) tidily from a container. This system, which you assemble yourself, has one important advantage over the dispenser: you can filter the substance as you extract it from the bottle or canister. This is important when DMSO is used orally (as a drink) or when it is applied intravenously.

All you need for this extraction appliance is a piece of PTFE tube with an inner diameter of 3 to 4 millimetres and a Luer lock adapter that fits the tube. The tube is inserted into one end of the adapter and a standard plastic medical syringe can be firmly attached to the other. This small adapter is called a 'female Luer lock'. The tube only needs to be as long as the container is high so that it rests on the bottom and has a short length protruding from the fastener at the top.

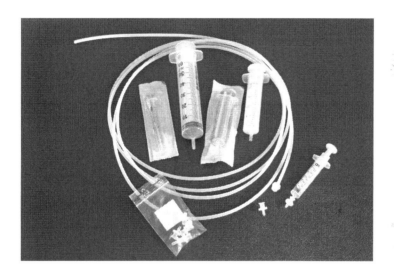

Figure 12: PTFE tube, Luer adapter and syringes

Place the adapter onto one end of the tube and drill a hole the size of the tube's external diameter in the seal of the DMSO bottle. If you do not know the external diameter you should measure it beforehand using a normal calliper. Use a clean tool to drill the hole, and drill a hole that is slightly too small. The open end of the tube is then pushed as far as possible through the cap (that is put back on) until it is almost sitting at the bottom of the container. Then attach a Luer syringe in the size of your choice onto the adapter, and cleanly extract the quantity you need.

You should then seal the system tightly either by closing it with a plug that fits tightly or by reattaching the emptied syringe. Luer syringes are available in standard sizes from between 1 and 60 millilitres and you can find an appropriate size for almost any purpose. The total cost of the accessories comes to a few pounds, although you usually have to buy a few metres of prepackaged tubing and standard multi packs of syringes.

Perhaps you know a doctor, alternative health practitioner or pharmacist who could give you single syringes. PTFE tubes are also commonly used in scientific and pharmaceutical laboratories, as well as in aquariums and in the motor trade.

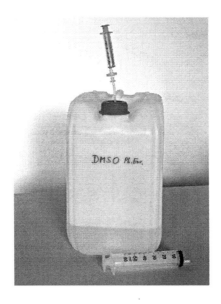

Figure 13: Container with extraction system and filter

As already explained in the section on 'Physical properties', DMSO's freezing point stands at around 18.5 °C. This means that the liquid becomes solid at temperatures slightly below normal room temperature (usually about 20 °C). DMSO is often delivered in a frozen state during the colder (European) seasons and it sometimes freezes when temperatures drop overnight. You should always keep it warm – above 19 °C – if you intend to use it. If it does become solid, you will need to warm it to above its freezing point since it must be in liquid form before it can be used. To do this, simply place it on a radiator overnight.

DMSO becomes solid

If you intend to prepare aqueous dilutions or to combine DMSO with other medicines, you should have suitable containers such as brown glass bottles, glass beakers or porcelain egg cups at the ready. You can then fill these with the required amount of DMSO using a pipette, syringe or dispenser. The quantity of water required for an aqueous dilution can be measured using a graduated cylinder, or you can draw up the water using a graduated pipette / syringe before adding it to the DMSO.

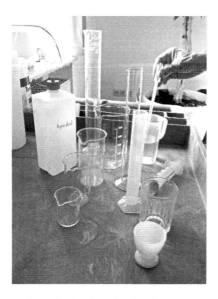

Figure 14: Graduated cylinder, glass beakers, egg cups, pipettes

Warning: As soon as you mix water and DMSO, a significant amount of energy in the form of heat is released – the solution and its container become noticeably warmer. This has to do with the molecular inter- *Heat* action that was explained in detail in the chapter on 'Scientific aspects' *generation* and is an example of what is known as an exothermic mixing reaction or solution reaction. This is a clear indication that both substances greatly influence one another and that they cannot subsequently be regarded as pure substances. Patients often say that the mixture, when used externally directly after it is produced, feels very pleasant. There is no reason why you must wait for the passively warmed solution to cool before use.

For smaller quantities, it is more practical for the mixture to be produced in the syringe by drawing both liquids into it one after the other, and then tilting the syringe a number of times to mix the solution. You can prepare even smaller quantities (less than 1ml) to treat scars, for example, by counting drops using a Pasteur pipette. The relevant details are given in the respective instruction sections.

Water that is used to dilute DMSO should be as low-germ as possible. Normal tap water can, of course, be used for applications on healthy skin. But since you may end up storing a freshly prepared solution for a long period of time, not knowing exactly when or for what reason you might eventually be using it, it is wise to establish good hygiene habits *Suitable* whenever you handle DMSO. The simplest solution is to buy deionised *water* water as used in steam irons and car batteries, and to boil it as you need it. Alternatively, you could use distilled, sterilised, filtered water that is intended for medicinal use. This can be bought in pharmacies and from medical practice suppliers. A third option is to use the sterile, isotonic sodium chloride solutions that are used for infusions and injections. Using such a mixture of sterile water and filtered DMSO you can treat wounds and administer nasal drops without worry.

We should at this point remind the reader of the possible side effects or physical reactions that can arise and are, to some degree, unwanted. As already explained in the first chapter, these reactions are actually closely related to the desired effects of DMSO.

Side effects These side effects include local reactions on the skin that vary from user to user. Comments by patients range from 'I don't feel anything!' to 'That feels like stinging nettles!' A common reaction is a rather pleasant tingling or pulsating feeling combined with minimal, local redness of the skin. Both these reactions usually disappear within a few minutes or hours. Generally speaking, people who have blonde or ginger hair and people who have low pigment concentration such as blue eyes, react slightly more sensitively to DMSO use. Morton Walker recommends using lower concentrations of DMSO when treating these groups of people.

It is very important not to surrender to the itching sensation and to irritate or damage the skin by scratching or rubbing the affected area during the period directly after applying the substance. It is wise to administer external applications during the day rather than just before going to bed because you are more likely to be distracted then. At night there is a risk that you might scratch the itchy skin in your sleep.

If the patient becomes very uncomfortable, adding more water or removing the DMSO solution from the skin using a damp cloth can provide instant relief. After one or more applications of the solution, the area of skin treated can temporarily become flaky, dry or rough. Such reactions will heal without treatment but, if you wish, you can apply small quantities of the most pure aloe vera product available. These reactions occur because DMSO, as a reliable 'carrier', transports the oils naturally present in the skin deeper into the body. The skin cells responsible must then work to produce a new protective surface layer.

Another very noticeable side effect of DMSO use is the well-known breath and body odour which lingers on many users soon after use. The reasons behind this odour were explained in detail in the first chapter. It is described by many as being similar to the smell of garlic or oysters. Personally, the smell reminds me of beached sea algae. Many people, particularly children, say it reminds them of 'Maggi' stock cubes. The differences in the way the odour is perceived are naturally dependent on the quantity of DMSO used. If you only treat a small scar locally then it is unlikely that anyone will notice any odour. Patients usually do not notice the smell because their nasal odour sensors become 'blind' to the sulphide compounds exuded.

Amusing situations often arise in crowded rooms (restaurants, for *Bear in mind* example) because other people often cannot identify an individual 'per- *the odour* petrator'. The only solution is to open the windows! You should bear this in mind if your work involves much contact with clients or customers, for example waiters or doctor's assistants. In that case you would need to decide what is more important. If necessary, treatment can be limited to weekends. Scientific evidence suggests that alcohol consumption can reduce the intensity of the DMSO odour. That is theoretically interesting because physiologically speaking they utilise the same liver enzyme system, but I cannot see that it would be possible to implement in practice. After all, there is little point in using a cytotoxin to undo the beneficial effects of DMSO.

It is always entertaining to hear stories by DMSO users regarding the *Amusing* inventive ways in which they solve such problems, and to listen to amus- *reports* ing reports concerning the reactions they have faced. I have heard of children who no longer want to be told bedtime stories, of married couples who decide to postpone trying to become pregnant, and of guests arriving at a country restaurant declaring that the place stinks to high heaven. Etiquette usually dictates that you do not say anything. I once carried out an experiment and intentionally drank a large quantity of DMSO on the day of a course I was teaching. Since I usually arrive early to prepare, there was no doubt that the place would smell by the time the participants arrived. Not a single one of the alternative medicine students commented on the smell until I brought up the issue myself. Most then agreed, saying that they had indeed been wondering the whole time what it might be. But some could not perceive the smell even when I told them about it. Everyone is different.

2.2 EXTERNAL ADMINISTRATION

Resorption

DMSO solutions can be applied externally both by moistening large areas of skin (cutaneous application) for the purpose of a general intake of DMSO, and by dabbing local areas of skin. Topical or local use (in contrast to systemic use through oral intake or infusion) can include administering drops into body orifices such as ears or nose. The distinction between topical and systemic applications of DMSO is never exact because DMSO penetrates all skin layers extremely quickly and can be detected in the blood very soon after being applied locally.

Research by K. H. Kolb[52] shows that traces of DMSO can be detected in human blood five minutes after 2 grams of the substance is applied cutaneously (on the skin). The values in the venous blood rise to a maximum level after 4–6 hours before slowly dropping again over the next 1–3 days. Even without the insights provided by such research we know that patients with skin lesions who bathe one hand in a DMSO solution also experience an improvement in the other hand, which was not treated locally. It indicates that DMSO, when applied externally, not only has an effect locally but also works systemically, i.e. in the whole body.

It is clear that the odour described above, which develops in most users, can also be perceived after external application if the quantity used is sufficient (or if the olfactory system is sensitive enough). A number of DMSO users take advantage of this property and apply large quantities of an appropriate dilution externally in order to avoid infusions, or to avoid drinking the substance. In my opinion, this is only wise if the skin can tolerate the DMSO solution well. If the skin becomes very itchy or red (this varies from individual to individual) and you find the reaction overly unpleasant then there is no need to torture yourself unnecessarily.

The first chapter cited a well-known clinical study on more than 100 American prisoners, some of whom had to drop out of the trial because of excessively severe skin irritation.

First-pass effect

It should be noted here that DMSO administered via the skin, and the same is true of DMSO administered via infusions, is not subject to the first-pass effect (as is the case regarding oral administration). All substances that enter the body via the digestive system (i.e. by drinking or eating) pass, via the portal venous system, through the liver during the first circulation in the bloodstream. The liver, as the most important metabolic organ, can then either immediately convert or break down these substances.

For many synthetic medicines this process results in a loss of efficacy that must be balanced by correspondingly higher doses. To the best of my knowledge there is no significant difference between DMSO levels in the blood after it is administered using any of the various methods (cutaneous, oral, intravenous), particularly since the most common way in which the substance is transformed is via the oxidation process that forms MSM, another medicinal substance (see Chapter 1.1 'What is DMSO?'). Besides, the half-life of DMSO and MSM in plasma is comparatively long. They can be detected in the blood for a number of days, suggesting that we need not worry about the liver's first-pass effect. Nevertheless, we can safely say that DMSO administration via the skin, and the same is true of DMSO administered via infusions, leads to the substance being fully available. In contrast, the DMSO contained in any solution you drink, like most foodstuffs you consume, will first have to pass through the liver.

Note: reactions when administering DMSO externally will usually be more severe above the waistline than below it. You may well find that local intolerances experienced when applying DMSO to skin on the torso or head do not occur when applying the substance to knees or ankles. Reactions such as redness, itching or burning are reversible and will subside within a short period of time. It is often the case that patients and users perceive the prickling and pulsating feeling as pleasant and warming, or that they associate the desired effects with these sensations. The extent of these reactions can be limited by rinsing the skin with pure water or by washing off the remaining DMSO using a damp cloth. Should you have used too much DMSO, causing a strong burning feeling, simply brush or spray additional water onto the affected area so that the remaining DMSO comes away as a highly diluted solution onto the cloth.

Warning: DMSO is an excellent solvent. That means it can quickly absorb a number of substances and carry them into the body with ease. This characteristic is used medicinally to transport other substances into deeper layers of tissue. Unfortunately this is not limited to beneficial substances – DMSO makes no distinction between good and bad. This is the reason why this book places so much emphasis on hygiene when *Precautionary measures* dealing with DMSO. Other issues may not be instantly obvious. For example, make sure that the materials from which containers and accessories (e.g. brushes and swabs) are made are not dissolvable, causing the ingredients to fall onto the skin. It is always best to use glass or ceramic containers. Plastic containers should always be made of HDPE.

You should also be fastidious in ensuring that clothing does not come into contact with the treated areas too soon after application.

DMSO quickly dissolves dyes, industrially applied textile finishing and washing agents from clothing, potentially causing allergic reactions. Redness of the skin and wheals that last for many days are often falsely attributed to DMSO when in fact they are caused by other chemicals. If it is not possible to wait until the DMSO has been completely absorbed by the skin before getting dressed, it is important to remove the remaining liquid from the skin using a damp cloth and only then should you get dressed again.

You should also ensure that DMSO does not find its way onto furniture such as treatment tables as it can dissolve the cushioning materials and the painted frames.

The following easy-to-find items have proven to be useful accessories when applying DMSO externally:
- wads of cotton wool
- porcelain egg cups
- soft hair brushes in various sizes
- brown glass bottles with droppers or pipettes
- white cloths / towels in various sizes that you do not bleach or soften when washing them
- kitchen rolls
- suitable mixing and dipping containers such as dessert bowls
- measuring accessories such as teaspoons, pipettes, syringes and graduated cylinders.

Basic mixture Taking a **tolerance test** is **always** the first step in any DMSO treatment. To do that you will need to prepare a standard aqueous solution of 70%. Depending on the total quantity you require, measure 30 parts water and 70 parts DMSO using a teaspoon, pipette, syringe or graduated cylinder, and place both liquids in a single container. To obtain the smallest possible quantity mix 7 drops of DMSO with 3 drops of water in an egg cup using a Pasteur pipette. You could also mix 7 teaspoons of DMSO with 3 teaspoons of water. **One teaspoonful is roughly equal to 3ml.** The teaspoon method gives a total quantity of about 30ml. Seven tsp. DMSO + 3 tsp. water (at 3ml each) totals 30ml.

To prepare exactly 10ml of a 70% DMSO solution, measure 3ml of water and 7ml of DMSO using a pipette, and then mix both liquids in a brown glass bottle or, if using the liquid immediately, in a small tumbler. To prepare 100ml, you will need 30ml of water and 70ml of DMSO.

The tolerance test is done by dabbing the 70% DMSO solution onto the crease of the elbow. You then observe this area and wait at least one hour, or preferably one whole day. If you experience a prolonged allergic reaction, liver pains or any other unpleasant symptoms you are advised against taking DMSO.

> **Note:** all containers used to store, mix and decant DMSO (or other substances) should be clearly labelled. Even though DMSO is a very safe substance you should still make certain that children, for example, do not drink it unknowingly. You will make life easier for yourself if you not only pay heed to good hygiene but also to orderliness. When you use bottles and glasses that were previously used to store other foods or substances it can become difficult to keep track of what each one is used for unless they are clearly labelled. You might also need to prepare and store different concentrations of aqueous DMSO solutions, in which case it really pays to record exactly what is in each container.

Once the mixture has been shaken or stirred, forming a homogenous solution, dip a wad of cotton wool into it and use it to dab a previously washed area of skin (in the elbow crease, for example). If over the next few minutes or hours you only feel a slight itching, a redness of the skin, or a prickling sensation, or if you feel nothing at all, then you can use DMSO. If a wheal or pustule develops immediately, or if the skin becomes red beyond the area treated, you should take care; wait for at least one hour, preferably one whole day, and then observe how the reaction develops. You might then choose to test a weaker solution (40 to 60%) *Suitable* or try treating only the skin below the waistline with DMSO. Over *solutions* time you will develop a certain instinct regarding which dilutions of DMSO can be effectively used to treat specific symptoms. Below are a few suggestions.

Administration of large quantities via the skin on the legs:	60 to 80% DMSO
Treating joints or muscles on the torso:	40 to 70% DMSO
Treating sports injuries to the arms and legs:	60 to 75% DMSO
Preparation of ear and nose drops:	25 to 50% DMSO
Solution prepared with sterilised water to treat open wounds:	30 to 60% DMSO
For dabbing warts:	80 to 90% DMSO

Other variations can be used depending on the relevant body part and individual tolerance. For example, Morton Walker recommends a DMSO preparation that contains only 5mg per millilitre of aqueous solution when treating the eyes. For that purpose mix 4.5ml of pure DMSO (= 4.95g) into a 1-litre infusion bottle of isotonic saline solution. It is a large total quantity but the process is far more practical than weighing milligrams, for which you would require a micro scale. The DMSO solution is then mixed, and drawn from the infusion bottle using a syringe and cannula.

Storage life All aqueous solutions have a long storage life as long as you pay attention to hygiene and cleanliness during the preparation process. If you forget to close a storage container there is no significant loss through evaporation. I often leave an egg cup filled with a prepared solution in the bathroom over a number of days because that is a good way to remember to take it. It should be noted, however, that DMSO vapour should not be inhaled because it changes the surface tension in the lungs. Since the boiling point of DMSO is very high (see Chapter 1.2.1 'Physical properties'), there is usually no significant or measurable vaporisation at room temperatures.

Now that you have made your first experiments with DMSO and have become familiar with the substance, let us take a closer look at exactly how it should be used externally.

Planning   Allow plenty of time for the application of DMSO. Bear in mind that it can take between 15 and 30 minutes for the solution to be completely absorbed when applied to the skin. If you intend to make repeated applications, it will take a correspondingly longer period of time before the skin is dry again. This application period is not relevant regarding some other modes of application such as using ear drops.

The same is true when the affected body area is not covered with clothing after DMSO application. In summer, when you are wearing shorts and a T-shirt, there is no reason why you should not carry on with your day brandishing a wet elbow. However, if you do so always make sure that the DMSO does not drip onto clothing, flooring (carpets, PVC, etc.) or furniture as it can cause damage. DMSO solutions are highly fluid, like water, and it is wise to take your time when applying them and not to apply too much. The following procedures have proven to be very useful for external application.

All clothing is removed from the affected body part and the patient sits *Brushing the* or lies down so that the affected area is easily accessible. The images *skin* below suggest how this can be done. Place white towels under or around the area being treated so that the solution does not trickle onto clothing, flooring or furniture.

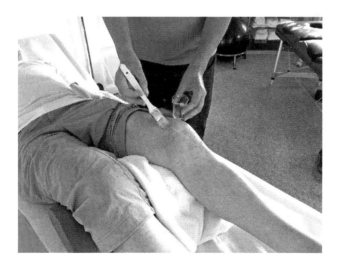

Figure 15: External DMSO treatment of the knee

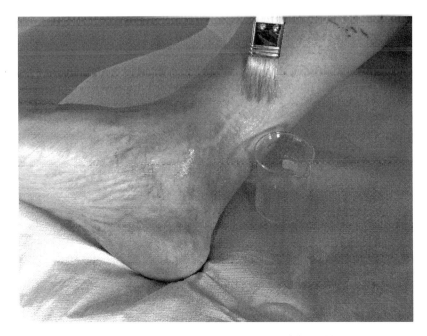

Figure 16: External DMSO treatment of the ankle

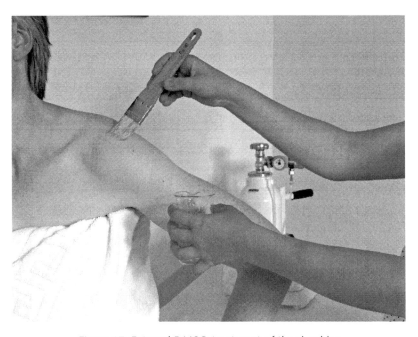

Figure 17: External DMSO treatment of the shoulder

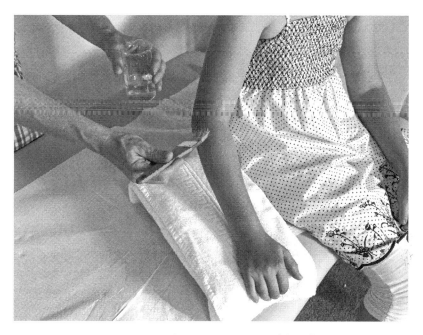

Figure 18: External DMSO treatment of the elbow

Clean the affected area of skin with a damp cloth (without soap) directly before the application of DMSO. Then dip the pad or brush into the DMSO solution (which you will have prepared in the correct ratio in advance), squeeze off the excess liquid on the edge of the container and brush the affected area extensively using criss-cross strokes so that the skin is well moistened.

To deliver DMSO into the body using external application, brush a 70 to 80% solution onto one or both legs repeatedly until the desired total quantity of DMSO has been applied. For example, using this method to apply a total of 20ml of an 80% solution onto the skin, the best-case scenario would be that about 17.5 grams of DMSO (density: 1.1g/ml) is absorbed, provided that no significant losses of liquid occur.

Spray bottles can be used as an alternative to brushing. They are available in a range of sizes, between 50 and 250ml. Hand-operated sprays, such as those used to care for houseplants, can be found in larger sizes. Always check that plastic bottles are suitable for use as DMSO containers. Materials that can be dissolved are unsuitable. Even if DMSO does not instantly create a hole in a plastic bottle, substances contained in some plastics can slowly dissolve into the liquid DMSO. This should be

DMSO as a spray solution

avoided at all costs because these substances, as explained above, are transported into the body when DMSO is applied externally. Bottles made of glass and HDPE are suitable for use as storage containers for DMSO.

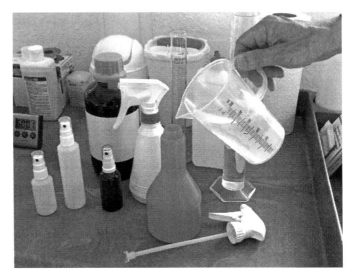

Figure 19: Spray bottles suitable for DMSO solutions

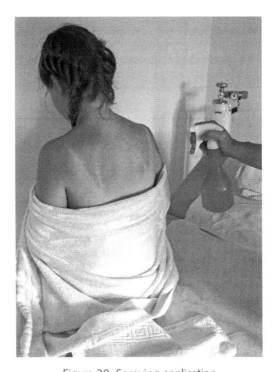

Figure 20: Spraying application

Note:
The spray drizzle of DMSO solutions must not be inhaled!

Spray solutions, in the recommended dilutions, are a suitable treatment for cuts or skin injuries. You should always use sterile water when preparing spray solutions and disinfect the spray bottle before use (e.g. using H_2O_2).

Allow 20 minutes for a single application of DMSO to be fully absorbed by the skin. After that period the area of skin will have dried and can be covered by clothing. However, if the patient has high tolerance, there is nothing to stop you from applying another dose of the solution when the skin has dried to some degree. You can repeat this several times but you will need to plan ahead. It would be a shame to have to end a treatment prematurely and wash off the DMSO because you need to be somewhere else by a certain time.

You can use basic cotton buds to dab DMSO onto small areas of skin, such as when treating warts. Even when applying small quantities, make certain that it has been completely absorbed by the skin before you cover the area with clothing.

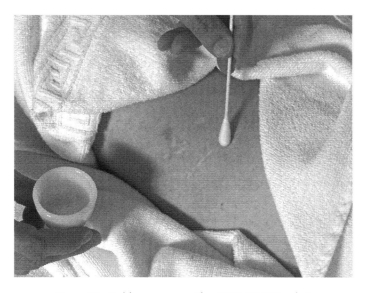

Figure 21: Dabbing a scar with a 70% DMSO solution

DMSO drops   Aqueous DMSO can also be used as ear and nose drops. Inflammation of the ear canal, blocked sinuses and other conditions can be treated in this way. The brown-glass dropper bottles that you need for this can be acquired from pharmacies or laboratory suppliers. They are available in sizes ranging from 5 to 250 millilitres. When using this method I prefer the 10ml bottles. If you need more, 20ml bottles can be used. However, since these drop solutions are prepared individually and usually yield the desired effect quite quickly you should not prepare too much unnecessarily.

When applying nasal drops start with low doses, i.e. prepare a weaker solution using water. The nasal membrane reacts sensitively and DMSO solution, in the first instance, often triggers an unusual tingling or even a burning sensation. Start with 2.5ml of DMSO in 10ml of solution (= 25%) and then increase when the user has become accustomed to it. For example, you can then put 3 or 4ml of DMSO into the 10ml brown-glass dropper bottle and top it up with sterilised water (= 30 to 40%). It is best to apply the drops while lying down so that you can apply 2 to 3 drops of the solution into each nostril comfortably. Then press the side of both nostrils with your fingers to close the nostrils; move them against one other to make certain the inner nostrils are well moistened. When treating sinusitis, only a few applications are needed before there is a clear improvement in the condition.

Ear drops are used to treat eczema and inflammations in the ear canal, along with a number of other conditions. The patient lies on his / her side and 1 to 2 drops of the prepared DMSO solution is put into the affected ear. The itching can increase for a short period because the substance improves blood circulation. As is the case for almost all types of external application of DMSO, you must 'grin and bear' the first few minutes and resist the urge to scratch the itch. You will hopefully be rewarded with a significant reduction in your symptoms.

The first scar   One of the images below illustrates the use of drops on the navel. The navel can be regarded as scar tissue and is a problematic area for many people. That is certainly true if the healing process was disrupted or if this 'gateway' was used during later, endoscopic operations / intrusions by means of surgical incisions. A number of health systems including traditional Chinese medicine (TCM) and yoga regard the navel as an important energy zone that needs care and attention. It is therefore good practice to treat the navel (again in a lying position) by applying a

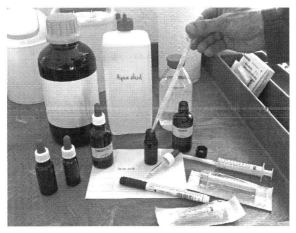

Figure 22: Dropper bottles suitable for DMSO solutions

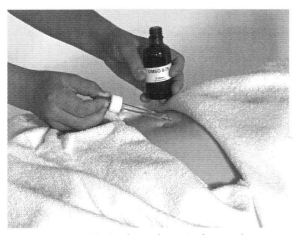

Figure 23: Applying drops to the navel

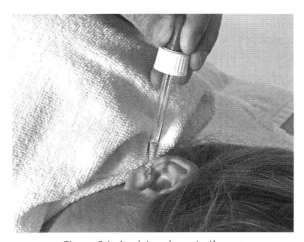

Figure 24: Applying drops to the ear

few drops of an aqueous DMSO solution and allowing it to be completely absorbed by the skin. Use higher concentrations when treating the navel because, unlike the membrane of the nose and ears, the skin here is not sensitive.

DMSO gel Many users prefer DMSO in gel form for external use so that it remains on the skin during the absorption period. Since the aqueous solutions that we have already discussed are naturally highly fluid, drops quickly form on the skin. Depending on which area of skin is being treated, the solution may flow onto towels. Long-lasting gels are produced industrially / pharmaceutically from raw materials such as polyacrylic acid derivatives. The process requires a certain knowledge and certain equipment (automated stirrers, pH-meters, etc.). It is, of course, possible to acquire these and I am surprised that such DMSO gels are not widely available on the internet. Personally I do not approve of the use of such raw materials in DMSO treatment. DMSO transports all other substances it is mixed with, into the body. Do you want to absorb synthetic materials?

One natural way of making a viscous DMSO preparation is to mix it with a pure aloe vera gel (at least 99.5%). The same dilution recommendations apply here as when preparing liquid solutions. A standard gel for external application contains about 70% DMSO and 30% aloe vera. The formula can be rounded off with a few drops of benzoin Siam. However, such mixtures can generally only be stored for short periods and should be freshly prepared and stored in a cool place if you intend to use them more than once.

2.3 ORAL ADMINISTRATION

If you are mainly aiming for a systemic administration of DMSO (i.e. providing DMSO to the whole body), drinking a diluted DMSO solution is a convenient alternative to applying it to large areas of skin. As explained in the previous chapter, the local treatment of specific areas of skin cannot be completely separated from systemic application because DMSO always penetrates the skin, making its way into all body tissue (except for hair and nails). Using external application, the total quantity of DMSO absorbed is decisive in terms of whether the patient enjoys a noticeable, holistic effect throughout the whole body. The chances of this happening are naturally greater when brushing the knee with generous quantities of DMSO than it is when treating a small scar or eczema locally / externally.

The 'first-pass effect' must be taken into consideration during oral administration. When substances are absorbed by the bowel, they are subject to a decomposition or conversion process in the intestinal wall or in the liver, organs the substance must pass through before entering the systemic circulation. This is true both for medications and for foods that are metabolised by the liver. Taking medications leads to an (unwanted) loss of the active substance because the liver, for example, attempts to improve the substance's water solubility and its excretability via the kidneys. One option that bypasses this effect is to use suppositories, plasters or injections. Otherwise the loss of efficacy must be made up for by increasing the dose, which is a common solution.

DMSO is only partially converted, becoming MSM, a sulfone that has valuable health benefits and which is a naturally occurring substance (see Chapter 1.1 'What is DMSO?').

An even smaller part (about 1%) is broken down, causing the infamous odour that can be detected after taking DMSO. The bioavailability of DMSO and its oxidation product MSM are comparable at around three days, meaning that the first-pass effect can be disregarded. That is the reason why the measurable metabolic rates after external application take a very similar course. After all, the liver has to attend to all the substances circulating in the blood and DMSO largely leaves the blood circulation at an early stage because it dissociates through all biological barriers and spreads through the body tissue.

Let us take another look at the question of how much DMSO should be *Dose* administered in systemic applications. Chapter 1.2.4 ('Safety of the medicinal product') presented the results of the clinical trial carried out on volunteers in 1967–68. Over a maximum period of 90 days these test subjects took 1 gram of DMSO per kilogram of body weight without any evidence of any toxic side effects. This means that a DMSO user weighing 70kg could take 70 grams of the substance every day. In my opinion this is rather unrealistic when it comes to external or oral use. Such doses can only be reasonably administered, if at all, intravenously in the form of a suitable infusion solution. However, that should only be given in particularly acute and severe cases, and then only by experienced professionals.

To take 70g of DMSO externally, the skin would have to absorb 100ml of a 70% solution. That would take a very long time and would probably cause severe skin irritation. Taking 70g of DMSO in drink form is not a particularly reasonable prospect either. Starting with such high doses is unnecessary because DMSO levels in the body (due to the long half-life) increase over a period of a few days if you continue taking it.

It is advisable to start taking DMSO at a low dose of about 3.5g in a glass of water and to observe the symptoms you are treating. If, for example, the joint or muscle pains are relieved and you appear to be tolerating the substance well, remain at that dose. If not, then increase the dose, for example in increments of 3.5g per day.

To prepare a drink solution, you will need appliances that can measure quantities of liquid DMSO more or less to the millilitre. Use pipettes and syringes, or use the measuring cups and spoons provided with other liquid medications. You can also use teaspoons: one teaspoon is roughly equal to 3ml.

DMSO tastes bitter when mixed with water. If that bothers you, add juice or cooled tea to improve the taste. Morton Walker recommends grape or tomato juice. There are bound to be other recommendations. Personally, I would not recommend tomato juice because we know that DMSO releases histamines from the body's cells. It is up to you to find a pleasing combination.

DMSO drink Pour the quantity of DMSO measured beforehand (e.g. 3.5g) into a glass (about 300ml). Then fill the glass with your chosen drink, making sure the two substances are mixed well. If you add DMSO to the glass after pouring the drink, the DMSO sinks to the bottom because of its higher density, causing the last 'gulp' to be extremely bitter. It is therefore important to stir it well. That gives you a 1 to 2% DMSO solution that should be easy to drink.

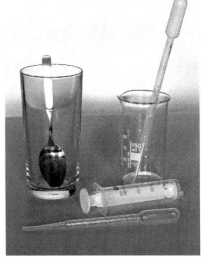

Figure 25: Measuring utensils used to prepare a drink solution

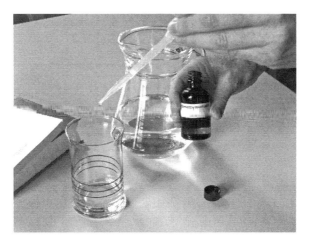

Figure 26: Preparing a measure of DMSO drink solution

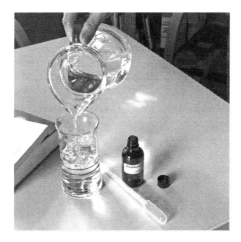

Figure 27: Topping up with water

Immediately after breakfast has proven to be a popular time to take DMSO. You can achieve equally good results by taking the DMSO solution at any other time of day, even taking it as and when you become aware of the symptoms you wish to treat. You should bear in mind that taking these quantities of DMSO has a diuretic effect. That means that more urine is produced in the first few hours after taking DMSO. Drinking the solution shortly before going to bed is therefore not recommended because the need to urinate will disrupt sleep. The same is true of taking DMSO just before important appointments or flights.

3.5ml of DMSO at a density of 1.1 gram per millilitre is equal to 3.85 grams. That gives you a dose of about 0.05g DMSO per kilogram of body weight if you weighed 75kg. These levels are still a long way away from the quantities that are labelled as being completely safe in most clinical trials and toxicity tests. You will remember that the volunteer prisoners were given 1 gram per kilogram of body weight for 90 consecutive days. That is 20 times these levels!

To achieve a stronger effect, increase the dose of DMSO; 7ml, twice the initial quantity, is equivalent to a dose of 0.1g per kilogram of body weight, etc. The only issues that might limit further increases in the dose would be the more intense taste and the possibility of causing slight irritation to the membranes of the throat. To take more than 10ml of DMSO per day (= about 300ml), it is recommended that you spread the dose over a number of drinks taken at different times of the day, for example after breakfast or before lunch.

2.4 ADMINISTRATION BY INJECTION

Permission Under German law, the self-responsible administration of intravenous infusions and the injection of such infusions under the skin (subcutaneous) or into the muscles (intramuscular) may only be carried out by doctors and alternative health practitioners. With regard to making independent diagnoses and choosing a treatment, these two professional groups are equal before the law – Germany is the only country in the world where this is the case. All other jobs in the health system are classed in the category of 'healthcare assistants' who may, strictly speaking, only take action if instructed to do so by a doctor or alternative health practitioner. Assistant roles include paramedics, nurses, physiotherapists, medical technologists and pharmacists (the word prescription comes from the Latin *recipe* – 'take it!'). Even if this legally anchored principle is often bypassed in practice, or the direction of the doctor or alternative health practitioner is tacitly assumed, it must nevertheless be mentioned here.

Becoming an alternative health practitioner Anyone who is interested in this profession and has the required mind-set has the option of training to become an alternative health practitioner, either at our institution *Praxisinstitut Naturmedizin* (www.Pra-Natu.de) in Germany or at another institution. Seek neutral and honest advice because there are certainly unsuitable study options available. Our students tell us that important factors to consider are a friendly, constant group of participants, professional and assured teachers who can soundly communicate the important basic information on anatomy and physiology, and an opportunity to deepen one's knowledge and understanding of individual treatments.

Along with acquiring permission to administer solutions intravenously, subcutaneously or intramuscularly, there is actually one other official prerequisite for this kind of administration. The relevant infusions or ampules must be approved by the authorities in accordance *Approval?* with the German Medicines Act.* Each type of application / use of a medication (and not only the medication itself) intended for humans and animals is subject to this approval requirement. Regarding DMSO, it is of little help that this substance is available in the (combination) preparations, creams and drops mentioned at the beginning, and that these applications have been approved. These are unsuitable for use by means of injection, and the bureaucratic 'blessing' cannot be transferred to DMSO in the form of an aqueous dilution.

These solutions cannot be prescribed, the cost is not met by health insurance providers, and they are used solely on the responsibility of the health practitioner and (private) patient.

The reasons why DMSO solutions have not been granted official approval are complex and, as explained in the introduction, must be understood within the political context of the pharmaceutical and healthcare industries. This is also the reason why veterinarians and doctors, especially when it comes to well-known figures, do not speak publicly about this method of DMSO use – not unless there is a close and trusting relationship.

Despite that, this healing substance is used as a matter of course in the private practices of well-known (sports) doctors, cosmetic surgeons, vets and alternative health practitioners. One of the most highly prized effects of DMSO is improved recovery times for 'precious' sportspeople, sport horses and other stars. If you research DMSO infusions, you will mainly find references to their use on sports horses. The topic is discussed relatively openly in this field.

Paravac, an emulsion having DMSO as its basis, was developed by the immunA company and there was talk of conducting Phase 3 clinical research on it. But it has all gone quiet again with regard to this substance, which unfortunately contained a whole host of controversial ingredients alongside DMSO. Among them were dimethicone (polydimethylsiloxane) and oil-based adjuvants, such as the ones used in

---

* News: As of November 2015 DMSO ampules are officially available in Germany!

supposed vaccination adjuvants. Personally I would never use such a mixture because I see no reason for bothering with preparations that include a number of unnatural chemicals. They are a mark of pronounced business interests, which are very different from the interests of truly independent health practitioners.

We should enjoy the fact that there is such a broad range of applications for pure DMSO mixed in the appropriate concentrations with pure or isotonic water. If people are not patient or flexible enough to use these natural liquids, perhaps we should be asking whether they are genuinely interested in alternative medicine.

Producing your own The fundamental problem with regard to the use of DMSO as an infusion or administered by injection is that no ready-to-use solutions are available because this method has not been officially approved.* Solutions that are directly administered into the blood or the tissue must fulfil certain prerequisites. Compliance with hygienic quality criteria is hugely important in the industrial preparation of what is known as parenteral medications (ampules, infusions, etc.) in accordance with international GMP guidelines. This is meant to ensure that such medications are as sterile and free of pyrogens as possible when bottled. Pyrogens are substances that cause fever when they are administered intravenously. These include not only microbiological impurities or organisms (bacteria, viruses, fungi, etc.) but also pyrogens of non-organic origin. This latter category includes microscopic particles formed during manufacturing processes as the result of the abrasion of plastics, metals or rubber. It is important that such substances do not enter the medication. Dilettantish experiments with impure substances have no place in the parenteral administration of medications.

The DIY production of infusion or injection solutions requires full compliance with basic hygiene rules to eliminate the risk of impurities entering the medication. Reports of 'allergic reactions' such as chills and shivering after being given infusions / injections can, in my opinion, often be traced back to a lack of knowledge regarding how to prepare these solutions. This is also true of infusions of MMS and other substances. It takes much effort to acquire the necessary expertise and experience for dealing with sterile liquids. If you cannot or do not want to do this work, it is best to seek the assistance of a doctor or alternative health practitioner who can demonstrate and explain all the necessary

* News: As of November 2015 DMSO ampules are officially available in Germany!

steps. Health practitioners could choose to have small quantities of in-fusions produced for them under GMP conditions. Some companies in this sector allow you to bring your own ingredients and to produce your own infusions under sterile conditions following their instructions.

Below are the minimum requirements for producing your own prep- *Minimum* arations for intravenous administration. *equipment*
requirements

First, you need a clean worktop such as a laboratory bench or a kitch-en worktop that you can sterilise with a surface disinfectant. When working with the materials wear a clean lab coat, face mask and single-use gloves. I recommend searching for a reliable laboratory or medical supplies company who can give you good advice.

To produce DMSO infusions you will need the correct raw materials, i.e. DMSO in certified pharmaceutical quality (Ph. Eur.). We can provide you with references to good suppliers upon request, or simply research the internet. If you, like me, are lucky enough to know people working in scientific research you may be able to have DMSO distilled under cleanroom conditions in a vacuum over sodium hydroxide, and have it bottled in a septum bottle in a protective atmosphere.

Otherwise you will have to work with sterile nanofilters, using them to purify DMSO before use in an infusion. This option was suggested indirectly within the instructions on how to assemble the DIY extraction *Syringe filter* appliance (Chapter 2.1). You will need individually packaged, sterile, and encapsulated syringe filters that have Luer connections on both sides. That allows you to use them as connectors with normal medical syringes. These should also be in sterile packaging and have a valid use-by date. Syringe filters are available in a variety of sizes, pore sizes and materials. Filters with pore sizes of 200 nanometers or less and with the filter material marked as PTFE (polytetrafluorethylene) or PA (poly-amide = nylon) are suitable. But it is best to ask the supplier what kinds are most suitable for filtering DMSO.

Before filtering, it is recommended that you heat the required quantity of DMSO to a temperature of between 70 and 90 °C to 'neutralise' any biological impurities that might be contained in it. This denatures micro-organisms and enzymes. To do this, pour the DMSO into clean, disinfec-ted laboratory glassware (glass beaker, Erlenmeyer flask) or a glass teapot, and heat it on the stove. I recommend monitoring the heating process by placing in the container a simple glass laboratory thermometer that has a suitable measuring range (e.g. -15 to +150 °C). Alternatively, the tempe-rature can be measured without contact using an infrared thermometer.

Caution: DMSO is flammable and its vapour is easily ignited. Do not heat the liquid on an open flame, do not overheat, and stay away from all sources of ignition!

Absolute cleanliness is an absolute must when preparing DMSO for administration!

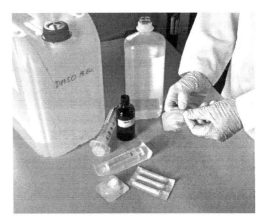

Figure 28: Material for the DMSO infusion

10 steps for preparing infusions If you do not want to assemble the extraction appliance as I recommended earlier, place a sterile injection cannula in front of the filter to extract DMSO from the bottle. It is absolutely vital that you throw this needle away after drawing DMSO from its container and that you use a new one to deliver the DMSO into the infusion bottle. Whichever method you use, you should proceed as follows.

1. Make sure the worktop is clean and sterile.
2. Have the following equipment to hand:
   - DMSO Ph. Eur. (preheated if possible)
   - sterile syringes / filters / cannula in appropriate sizes
   - infusion bottle(s) or bag(s) containing isotonic saline or electrolyte solution, 500 or 1000ml
   - waste container for used injection needles.
3. Wear a lab coat, face mask and single-use gloves.
4. Take a syringe of the desired size out of its sterile packaging.
5. Open the sterile packaging of the syringe filter then place the filter on the syringe with the female Luer lock.
6. Fit the male Luer lock or a syringe cannula (yellow, 20G) onto the extraction appliance.

7. Extract the required quantity of DMSO from the container, bringing it into the syringe through the filter.
8. Remove the cannula / filter from the syringe and fit a new cannula onto it.
9. Use the cannula to prick a hole in the rubber septum at the designated place on the neck of the infusion bottle and inject the DMSO into the infusion solution.
10. Swirl to mix the liquids in the infusion bottle.

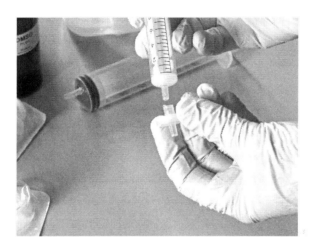

Figure 29: Fitting the sterile nanofilter

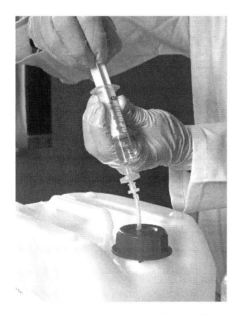

Figure 30: Draw up the DMSO through the filter

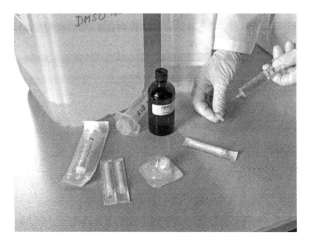

Figure 31: Remove the nanofilter

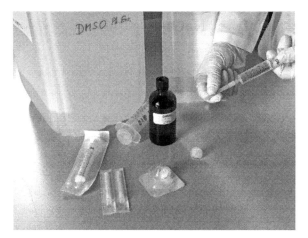

Figure 32: Fitting the sterile cannula

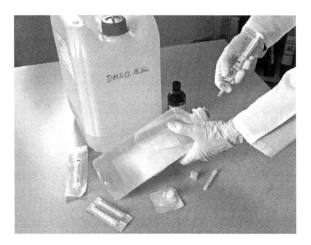

Figure 33: Injecting the purified DMSO through the septum

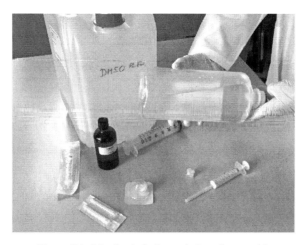

Figure 34: Mix the infusion solution thoroughly

Alternatively you could draw up the DMSO without a filter and then place the nanofilter between the cannula and the syringe before you inject it into the infusion solution. That is a matter of personal preference.

You will notice that it is quite difficult to push the viscous DMSO through these small-pore filters. To make this step a little easier mix the DMSO with a certain quantity of **sterile** water beforehand. For example, you could prepare a 25% DMSO solution by mixing 1 part DMSO with 3 parts water. The solution is more fluid than pure DMSO and does not require as much power when filtered. If you are using a 25% DMSO solution, administer four times as much in order to give the same total quantity of DMSO.

If you do not need to use the prepared infusion immediately, it should be stored away from light, for example in a cupboard.

Always bear in mind that these procedures are carried out on your own responsibility; you must consider whether these substances will be used only for self-treatment or whether others will also use them.

The DMSO infusion dose is based on body weight, in accordance with *Calculations* the guidelines given in the previous chapter section 'Oral administration'. When deciding on the dose make sure that the overall concentration of the solution is not too high, so as to avoid causing irritation to the veins. A solution of around 13% (vol. %) is usual for horses but remain well below this level when treating humans. If you weigh 70kg and want to infuse 0.2g DMSO per kilogram of body weight, then you will need 14g (about 12.5ml) of pure DMSO in the infusion bottle. If that is a 500ml electrolyte infusion, you will have a concentration of only 2.8% volume – well below 13%.

To administer more than 25ml of DMSO (= 27.5g) at any one time, I recommend using a 1000ml infusion. If you are concerned about administering large quantities of salt (NaCl) – 1 litre of an isotonic NaCl solution does contain 9 grams, after all – then you can use a 5% glucose infusion as an alternative.

The following table gives you an overview of what you need to know.

Conversion:

1ml DMSO = 1.1g DMSO → 1g DMSO = 0.91ml DMSO
1g/kg BW ≙ 1 gram per kilogram of body weight
10 ml DMSO:

in 250ml infusion solution → ≈ 3.8% vol. ≈ 4.2% weight
in 500ml infusion solution → ≈ 2% vol. ≈ 2.2% weight
in 1000ml infusion solution → ≈ 1% vol. ≈ 1.1% weight

50ml DMSO:

in 500ml infusion solution → ≈ 9% vol. ≈ 9.9% weight
in 1000ml infusion solution → ≈ 4.8% vol. ≈ 5.2% weight

When calculating the concentration level, bear in mind that the volume of DMSO added increases the total quantity of the infusion solution prepared. Use a simple calculation to work out the dilution you have in terms of volume or weight percentage, depending on whether you are basing the dose on millilitres or grams. The calculation below is based on the example of an infusion bottle filled with 500ml of electrolyte solution, topped up with 50ml of DMSO.

50ml DMSO ≙ x%
550ml total ≙ 100% → x% = (50 ml • 100%) / 550ml = 9.1% vol.

To calculate in terms of weight percentage, the DMSO volume in millilitres must first be multiplied by the density of 1.1g/ml. We will assume the density of the aqueous infusion solution to be 1g/ml. Using the above example, the formula would look like this:

55g DMSO ≙ x%
555g total ≙ 100% → x% = (55g • 100%) / 555g = 9.9% weight

DMSO infusions can be administered at relatively fast drop rates. In *Drop rate* contrast to the oxidant ClO_2 (the effective substance in MMS), for which the transporting vehicles such as the red blood cells and other carriers have limited capacity, DMSO dissolves extremely well in the blood even in high quantities and has a high distribution speed. As is the case with high-dose ascorbic acid infusions, it is desirable to flood the body with relatively high levels of DMSO. A 500ml infusion at doses based on the above guidelines can be administered at a rate of 300 drops per minute so that it is finished in about 30 minutes.

We will now discuss **subcutaneous** or **intramuscular** injections of aqueous *10 steps for* DMSO solutions. The concentration of the previously prepared dilution *preparing* must be taken into consideration. The same hygiene and sterilisation rules *injections* must be observed when preparing these applications as is the case for infusions. The most important difference is the total volume of the injection solution, which, in contrast to the infusion, is only a few millilitres.

Below is the preparation process.

1. Make certain that the worktop is clean and sterile.
2. Have the following equipment to hand:
   - DMSO Ph. Eur. (preheated if possible)
   - sterile syringes / filters / cannula in appropriate sizes
   - ampules or injection bottles containing isotonic saline solution
   - perhaps a mini-spike to allow access to the injection bottle
   - waste container for used injection needles.
3. Wear a lab coat, face mask and single-use gloves.
4. Take a syringe of the desired size out of its sterile packaging.
5. Open the sterile packaging of the syringe filter then place the filter on the syringe with the female Luer lock.
6. Fit the male Luer lock onto the extraction appliance or fit an injection cannula (yellow, 20G) onto the male Luer lock.
7. Swiftly draw up the required quantity of DMSO from the container, bringing it into the syringe through the fitted filter. Ensure that there is sufficient space in the syringe for the sterile water that must be added later.
8. Remove the cannula / filter from the syringe and place the syringe on the mini-spike in the injection bottle containing isotonic saline solution, or fit a new cannula, with which you can draw up the NaCl solution from a previously opened ampule.

Continue filling the syringe with the sterile saline solution up to the desired total volume.

9. Remove this cannula too from the syringe or pull the syringe out of the mini-spike, then swirl the liquids in the syringe to mix thoroughly.

10. Place the cannula that is suitable for your intended purpose on the syringe. Shorter needles with smaller diameters are normally used for subcutaneous injections (e.g. violet or blue, 24/23G), while stronger / longer needles are used for intramuscular injections (e.g. black or green, 22/21G).

Similar considerations arise regarding DMSO concentrations when injecting and when preparing infusions. If you fill a 5ml syringe, following the above steps, with 1ml DMSO and 4ml isotonic saline solution, you obtain a 20% solution in terms of volume.

1ml DMSO $\hat{=}$ x%
5ml total $\hat{=}$ 100% → x% = (1ml • 100%) / 5ml = 20% vol.

For subcutaneous or intramuscular injections in general, higher concentrations can be used than that used in infusions administered directly into the blood circulation. In principle, these injections should be regarded as local or topical administration, in contrast to the systemic application of infusions. However, as has already been explained, local and systemic applications cannot be strictly separated because DMSO quickly diffuses throughout the whole body in both cases. Looked at in this way, intramuscular injections replace or reinforce brushing external (percutaneous or transcutaneous) applications onto the same area. There is no significant difference in terms of the way in which the substance is distributed or excreted, for example via the urine, than is the case for the other application methods. The injection solutions used should contain (locally) effective concentrations of DMSO. For suggestions see the overview in Chapter 2.2.

2.5 DMSO ADMINISTRATION IN COMBINATION
WITH OTHER SUBSTANCES

'Combination preparation' is the term given to any medication that is produced by mixing at least two different substances for therapeutic use. This process is widely used and is intended to promote the synergistic properties of the individual substances. Admittedly, if you look at the shelves in any pharmacy you will see plenty of absurd substance combinations. Such products are usually only created for marketing reasons and so that the company can sell the product as 'new' and revolutionary.

When administering more than one substance at the same time there is a risk that when effects or side effects occur, it is impossible to know which of the ingredients was responsible. You do not know exactly which 'wheel' in the organism you have just turned. Using this method is therefore often worthless in terms of evaluating the efficacy of individual substances. In terms of the holistic search for the cause of disease by listening to the body's response to the therapeutic measures undertaken, it is of even less value. It could be countered that we often employ a number of very different household remedies to cure feverish colds, cuts and wounds, or musculoskeletal injuries. In such cases, drawing *Good reasons* from past experience, we treat our bodies using combinations of heat, *for* light, rest, poultices, water, prayer and a number of other 'medications' *combinations* without ever being able to 'prove' which was the most effective. Such confirmation is not necessary because we intuitively know that the synergy of the various substances has been beneficial for body, mind and soul.

Looking even more closely, we notice that we not only use various substances, but we also draw from the various properties and modulations that these substances possess. We are in fact discussing combinations of combinations.

When using DMSO as a single medicine we are already acquiring a combination of many different pharmacological effects.

Despite that, there are many good reasons why we should administer DMSO in combination with other substances. The most common of these is the desire to amplify the efficacy of medications that can penetrate more deeply into the tissue when they are dissolved in DMSO. In my opinion, before trying such a combination, you should already have carried out at least one DMSO-only administration to observe any reactions and to ensure that you tolerate the substance well. Only then can you assess the need for a DMSO combination, and subsequently evaluate its effect. If, in cases of acute illness, time is limited and the 'full force' of an effective treatment must be employed urgently, you can implement immediately the proven combinations regarding which we have plenty of experience. Work on the deeper cause once the pain is relieved or the swelling has begun to subside.

2.5.1 DMSO and MMS / CDS or hydrogen peroxide

Read about MMS / CDS in Dr Antje Oswald's *The MMS Handbook: Your Health in Your Hands*. MMS is a defined sodium chlorite solution that is activated directly before use by lowering the pH value – this produces chlorine dioxide, which is a powerful oxidant. This treatment method was made popular by the American Jim Humble, who has achieved amazing results treating infections and tumours. That is why this method quickly established itself across the globe. In terms of chemistry and physiology, it can be placed in the 'bio-oxidative processes' category, with ozone therapy. Other 'relatives' include hyperbaric oxygen therapy, singlet oxygen therapy and the use of hydrogen peroxide. The following section gives useful information on the use of combinations of the antioxidant DMSO with oxidants, namely MMS / CDS (ClO_2) or hydrogen peroxide (H_2O_2).

The basics of oxidation Looking through the lens of evolution, we can say that one of the most significant biochemical achievements of the human body (together with other mammals and higher animals) is its ability to work with oxidative processes, and using them with great skill. It is a miracle that we feel comfortable in an atmosphere that is rich with oxygen (21% vol.).

That is because oxygen (O_2), from a chemical point of view, is a rather aggressive substance having a maximum positive oxidation potential of 1.23 volt (depending on pH value).[53] Ozone (O_3), which is an even stronger oxidant and is toxic for humans when inhaled, has a maximum oxidation potential of 2.07 volts.

In comparison, chlorine dioxide (ClO_2), the effective substance in activated MMS solutions, is a comparatively moderate oxidant with a maximum oxidation potential of 1.5 volts. This fact helps us to understand the oxidative selectivity of MMS / chlorine dioxide solutions, which ensures that the body tissue of the patient being treated remains undamaged. This is an important difference between MMS and mainstream chemotherapy medications. Or, to refer back to the introduction, MMS treatment does **not** cause hair loss or any other unpleasant side effects.

As the name suggests, anaerobes (which include a number of pathogenic microorganisms e.g. viruses, bacteria, fungi, etc.) cannot tolerate oxygen, which is vital for humans and which works oxidatively. Anaerobes are destroyed and made inactive in oxygenated atmospheres or by other oxidants (e.g. MMS / CDS, H_2O_2, ozone, etc.) because they are insufficiently equipped to survive in surroundings that have an oxidizing effect. Looking through the lens of evolution, we can say that these microorganisms were on Earth at a much earlier time, long before there was oxygen in the atmosphere. Therefore they had no reason to adapt to it. *Fighting infections*

Today we divide all (cellular) creatures into three domains: the Archaea, the Bacteria, and the Eukaryotes (the latter category includes all creatures whose cells have true nuclei, including humans). The Archaea and the early Bacteria (anaerobes) are, however, the eldest ancestor species of the higher animals and they paved the way for plants and animals. Oxygen was first released into the world's atmosphere because flora developed and used the process of photosynthesis (a well-known metabolic process whereby carbon dioxide, water and light are taken in and oxygen is expelled).

Because some of the various bacterial microorganisms are among our natural enemies today (i.e. are potentially pathogenic), we should not despise them utterly. Their appearance on Earth billions of years ago first created the conditions on this planet that we know and treasure today.

If they proliferate too aggressively in our bodies, leading to infections and symptoms of disease, they can be fought off naturally using oxidation. They are not sufficiently equipped with protective enzymes for this chemical process in the same way that higher animals (Eukaryotes) are. This is also true of bacteria that have by now become accustomed to oxygen (facultative aerobes), and those that even need oxygen (aerobes), as well as viruses, protozoans or parasites. They will all be destroyed by substances that have a higher oxidation potential than oxygen.

The trick is to use these oxidative substances in a way that will cause as little damage to the body's own cells as possible. This has been done for some time in ozone therapy, for example, but has now been taken to new levels by Jim Humble and his discovery of MMS.

Armed with this basic information, we can now put together the pieces of the biochemical jigsaw which science has provided us with. Higher animals such as humans have learnt over the course of evolution to cope with the 'oxidative pressure' of Earth's atmosphere. But that is not all. The human body has developed in highly unique ways and uses a number of oxidation reactions for metabolic processes – that is the true crowning achievement of our immune system's defence against disease.

Our immune system (i.e. the white blood cells – leucocytes) deploys strong oxidant substances in the continuous battle against intruders and *Natural* mutants (microorganisms or tumour cells). These substances include *immune* (hydrogen) peroxide, hypochloride, peroxynitrite (OONO-) or radical *defence* derivatives of other oxygen compounds (ROS) – all rather aggressive sounding 'ammunition'. Leucocytes use the extremely destructive potential of these molecules in immune defence mechanisms. Hydrogen peroxide and hypochloride belong within the permanent arsenal of the white blood cells, which use them to eliminate 'suspicious' particles. Hydrogen peroxide is formed from the even more aggressive superoxide (O_2-) with the aid of the enzyme superoxide dismutase (SOD). This enzyme is useful to all aerobic beings because it 'deactivates' the superoxide anions that, as a source of oxidative stress, can cause cell damage.

Oxidants, mainly free radicals, are therefore very important for the functioning of the whole body. The hydroxyl radical (HO·), for example, is able to 'burn' viruses, bacteria, tumour cells, fungi etc. due to its high oxidation potential of 2.3V. These substances help our scavenger cells, natural killer cells, and other members of the non-specific immune defence, to finally destroy the pathogens that have been detected or even 'detained'. This takes place by means of a process called lysis: the cell walls are perforated causing the whole cell to disintegrate.

It is by no means enough to phagocytise (eat up) the enemy whole because he could then attack the defence cell from the inside or breed and multiply within. No, it takes much more work than that: the adversary must be broken down into waste parts that are as non-hazardous as possible so that they can then be further metabolised or excreted. During the course of this ultimate battle to destroy bacteria, some of the phagocytes (scavenger cells) selflessly perish. Pus is then formed, which is a mixture of bacterial waste and expended white blood cells.

Incidentally, such discoveries form part of the research work carried out by the three winners of the Nobel Prize in Medicine in 2011. In the case of Ralph Steinmann, who died a few days before the ceremony, this distinguished prize was awarded posthumously for the first time. We now know from the results of Steinmann's work and that of others that, in terms of the fundamental work of the defence cells that detect and fight 'foreign' elements, it is irrelevant whether these are bacteria, viruses, fungi, degenerate tumour cells, toxins, pollen or any other antigens.

I am particularly happy to emphasise that at this point, because the pharmaceutical industry and those who speak on its behalf are always ready to put forward the argument that it is sheer idiocy to use the one and the same substance (MMS, DMSO) to treat such a variety of diseases as infections (viruses, bacteria, etc.), autoimmune processes (autoantibodies) or malignant tumours (mutated cells).

Our immune systems, however, perceive all these 'suspicious outsiders' as fundamentally similar triggers that activate the immune response.

Today it is increasingly suspected that a number of these diseases, in- *Infections as* cluding metabolic diseases, are caused by virus or bacterial infections *the cause* that the patient has suffered in the past. These infections may have occurred decades earlier and the patient might have no recollection of it because at the time they did not experience any of the typical symptoms such as fever or pain. It is now almost conventional wisdom that the autoimmune illness diabetes mellitus type 1, neurodegenerative diseases such as dementia, Parkinson's or multiple sclerosis, and various types of cancer, can be attributed to such past virus infections where the immune system was possibly unable to conquer the disease.

Increasing evidence from medical research indicates that various diseases which today come under strictly divided specialist disciplines can very likely be prevented using very similar means. There is an urgent need for effective treatment that is mainly focused on the (oxidation) deficiencies of the natural immune defence or on (temporary) weaknesses of that system. These discoveries are not new. They have been made by prize-winning medical researchers and – coincidentally – they explain the amazing effects of DMSO, MMS & Co.

This contrast between oxidatively robust and oxidatively sensitive *Safe capture* beings gives the impression that the world has, very practically, been divided into good and bad camps. But there is one thing that should be borne in mind. As useful as oxidative, chemical forces may be for immune defence functions, the body's own 'disinfection chemicals' such as peroxide or hypochloride must be kept in check. This is the real evolutionary achievement! Just as our body is able to cope with the exact quantity of oxygen set by nature without suffering oxidation damage, it must also be able to safely manage the other oxidants it produces as ammunition. This requires a high level of selectivity in two ways. Firstly regarding the quantities of substances formed: it is well known that too much or too little oxygen is harmful. Secondly, regarding the safety mechanisms that ensure that these aggressive substances can be caught and decomposed: this usually happens enzymatically, i.e. with the aid of special catalysts for the individual chemical decomposition reactions.

Safety mechanisms   This is where the antioxidants come to the fore. As is apparent from the name, these are substances that can neutralise aggressive oxidative compounds, or that can cause these compounds to be excreted in a safe manner. There are many antioxidant substances. You probably know the term from advertisements for nonprescription medications or dietary supplements. We are continuously being urged to consume more antioxidants or to daub our skin with them. They include well-known substances such as ascorbic acid (vitamin C), tocopherols (vitamin E), beta-carotene (provitamin A), flavonoids and glutathione. Considering the information presented above, you must decide whether it actually makes sense to consistently cancel out the oxidative substances we use to fight illnesses by taking antioxidants.

You may know that cancer patients are instructed not to drink coffee! Coffee contains a number of antioxidants! Tumour cells should actually be scavenged and destroyed by the defence cells of the non-specific immune system (phagocytosis **and** lysis). They are destroyed using oxidation – it has been scientifically proven that antioxidants can slow this process down. So it is worth considering whether giving the antioxidant industry your money is a wise choice.

This issue should be analysed in more detail because the various antioxidants work selectively. Nevertheless, we should be happy to discover that nature has equipped us with the necessary antioxidant mechanisms that allows the body to use and to extinguish aggressive, oxidative chemicals.

To summarise: as higher animals, we can deal with oxidants and we use them for metabolic processes and in the internal battle against diseases. These processes always run as a matter of routine and in a regulated way without us being consciously aware of them. We know, for example, that cell mutations occur in the body with statistical regularity a few times per week. It is thanks to the oxidative activities of the defence cells, which immediately destroy such 'suspicious' activity in the healthy body, that such mutations do not usually develop into a cancer or that not every intruding pathogenic bacteria causes an infectious disease.

So what is the point of haphazardly taking tablets that the advertisements inform us will have an antioxidant effect? The normal processes described above sometimes spiral out of control when the natural balance between oxidative and antioxidant processes is disturbed. In such cases it is possible to suffer excess oxidative stress because alcohol, cigarettes, pathogens, dietary habits or lack of exercise lead to a lack of antioxidants or to excess oxidant production.

The so-called diseases of civilisation develop because the normal repair and detoxification processes of the tissue are overburdened. Infections and low metabolic performance occur when there is a long-term lack of oxidants. Joint complaints, atopic problems, and digestive and neurodegenerative diseases arise where there is a long-term lack of antioxidants. That is why alternative medicine practitioners, when faced with such cases, work by administering the missing substances, as indicated by the symptoms. This chapter concerns three of these substances.

MMS / CDS works as a selective oxidant and is therefore able to make up for the deficits in oxidation power that have led to the unchecked propagation of pathogenic microorganisms (e.g. malaria parasite) or to the uncontrolled growth of abnormal cells (e.g. malignant cancers). Since the body's own immune system is clearly too weak to fight off the disease, when you take MMS / CDS you are imitating the oxidative capabilities of healthy defence cells. The MMS / CDS gives the immune cells a helping hand with the 'killing' work so that the body has only the 'cleaning up' work to do. As explained above, this affects all antigens, i.e. all foreign, pathogenic particles, cells and molecules. *Pro-oxidation*

In contrast, DMSO is a very useful antioxidant. It works selectively; this means that it does not intercept any oxidants arbitrarily. We therefore need not worry that taking it will weaken the effect of the oxidative MMS, as we think might be the case with vitamin C. DMSO most notably 'deactivates' the hydroxyl radicals (HO·) that it chemically catches. They, along with hydrogen peroxide and other reactive oxygen species (ROS), are formed in rather small quantities within the framework of the respiratory chain in the tissue. This occurs in the mitochondria (the energy centres of the cells), where oxygen and glucose are used to produce energy, reacting and forming water and carbon dioxide. Hypoxia (a lack of oxygen in the cells) is one of the main causes of the increased production of hydroxyl radicals. There can be a number of reasons for the reduced supply of *Antioxidation* oxygen to the cells. Some common causes include circulatory insufficiency (arteriosclerosis), sleep apnoea, anaemia or iron deficiency, nutrient deficiency, accumulation of poisons, or other diseases.

Intelligent combination   It will now be clear why it is worth treating a number of health problems using a combination of the antioxidant DMSO and an oxidant such as MMS / CDS (ClO$_2$) or hydrogen peroxide. DMSO works to capture harmful hydroxyl radicals in the undernourished and diseased tissue, and as a 'transporter' for improved diffusion of the oxidant that is dissolved in it. The oxidant, for its part, supports the immune system in the fight against harmful cells and particles; it does so by means of oxidative attacks that damage the cell walls of the bacteria or tumour cells. Both treatment approaches – pro-oxidation and antioxidation – are highly effective in their own right but when combined they mutually reinforce one other.

You will find an excellent description of the beneficial effects oxidants such as MMS / CDS and H$_2$O$_2$ have on the human body and its immune defence in Dr Antje Oswald's *The MMS Handbook: Your Health in Your Hands*. In that book she quotes from a summary of scientific findings by Thomas Lee Hesselink on this topic. One result that emerges clearly is that oxidants improve the diffusion of oxygen from the red blood cells into the tissue. The oxygen itself then works in the cells as an oxidant to produce energy by burning glucose. The oxygen is also used in detoxification, regeneration and immune processes. This gives weight to the recommendation that DMSO and oxidants such as MMS / CDS or H$_2$O$_2$ should be used together because the positive properties of the oxidants are more effective in combination with DMSO.

We could go into more detail regarding the biochemical mechanisms here because it really is a matter of electron transfer and oxygen equivalents, but Chapter 2 is intended to be mainly about the practical aspects of DMSO use. However, I did want to make it clear why the parallel use of what appear to be counteractive substances is appropriate in this case. You will have to forgive me for the occasional digression.

Comparison of oxidants   Below is a table listing the calculated oxidation potential achieved in a neutral solution (pH = 7). This will give you an overview of the 'oxidative power' of the various oxygen-containing substances. The standard potentials (ϵ_0) of the substances listed in the research literature[53] have been converted using the modified Nernst equation. It should be noted that the oxidative aggressiveness of the substances listed in this table is tamed when the pH value of the aqueous solution in which they are dissolved is raised. The pH value indicates how acidic the solution is. Values above 7 indicate increasingly alkaline substances, values below 7 indicate increasingly acidic substances. The solution reacts neutrally at a value of 7. Blood (which is an aqueous solution of substances) in the human body has a pH value of around 7.3, meaning that we are in the slightly alkaline zone.

Here is the formula:

$$\varepsilon_7 = \varepsilon_0 - 0.05916 \cdot pH \quad \leftarrow \quad pH = 7$$

Symbol	Common name	Standard potential ε_0	Ox. Potential ε_7
O ·	Atomic oxygen	2.4V	2.0V
HO ·	Hydroxyl radical	2.3V	1.9V
O_3	Ozone	2.1V	1.7V
H_2O_2	Hydrogen peroxide	1.8V	1.4V
HOCl	Hypochlorous acid (MMS 2)	1.5V	1.1V
ClO_2	Chlorine dioxide (MMS/CDS)	1.5V	1.1V
O_2	Oxygen	1.2V	0.8V
DMSO	Dimethyl sulfoxide	0.75V	0.3V
Vitamin C	Ascorbic acid = antioxidant!	− 0.04V	− 0.8V

Table 2: Oxidation potential of important substances

This mathematical / theoretical approach to the principles of oxidation therapy does not accurately reflect the actual circumstances within the body. We should probably accept that we will never know what really happens 'in there' between the medications we choose to use, and the blood cells, antigens, and cell surfaces. Measuring potentials in test tubes (in vitro) is not a true measurement of the processes that take place in the blood (in vivo). The oxidation potential of chlorine dioxide is usually only estimated at 0.9V under such conditions.

The two oxidants that Jim Humble introduced to the world of alternative medicine (MMS / CDS and MMS 2) are quite mild oxygen carriers. Under pH conditions similar to those found in human / animal blood, ClO_2 (MMS / CDS) is a 'soft' and very selective oxidant (electron acceptor). Conversely, we can assume that chlorine dioxide will act more aggressively in acidic surroundings (e.g. tumour tissue).

According to the table, hydrogen peroxide has a significantly higher maximum oxidation potential than oxygen. Its therapeutic use has also been the subject of extensive research in the past. I have already mentioned the work of the Texan researcher J. W. Finney, who studied the beneficial effect that combinations of DMSO and hydrogen peroxide can have on oxygen supply to the myocardial muscle.[43] Unfortunately, hydrogen peroxide has met a similar fate to that of other medications discussed in this book. Over the years, results from a number of research projects are gathering dust for the simple reason that no one, for varying reasons, will become rich from selling these substances.

This is also the case with MMS 2, or aqueous hypochlorous acid (HOCl). In the past, this substance was used successfully by doctors in thousands of cases, including in the treatment of acute injuries and wounds. I have already explained the importance of this hypochloride as ammunition for our white blood cells (defence cells). If nature has given us this oxidative substance to use in the battle against infections and cancer cells, we can legitimately ask why the authorities and the pharmaceutical industry are trying their best to sabotage and undermine Jim Humble's rediscovery of this medication.

We should remind ourselves of one important fact from the section 'What is DMSO?' before we proceed to examine the combination formulas: DMSO itself can be oxidised!

When one oxygen atom is transferred, MSM (or dimethyl sulfone) is formed, which is often called 'organic sulphur'. This substance is also used medicinally but, as you might expect, it does not display the biochemical properties that one would expect from the production of a solution of other medications. Therefore the aqueous preparations of the oxidants (MMS 2 or hydrogen peroxide) should either be diluted appropriately, or their preparation and administration should be carried out quickly, as Jim Humble recommends. After dilution, the next issue that may need to be considered is the prior pH value adjustment of the liquid solution because the oxidative power of MMS and hydrogen peroxide is weaker in the neutral zone. A third convenient option is 'staggered combination': first administer DMSO so that it is already distributed and present in the body tissue, then administer the oxidative substance after a short delay. This leads to a physiologically determined dilution, and the regulation of the pH value of both substances.

Let us proceed to look at concrete instructions regarding how to mix DMSO with suitable oxidants. Bear in mind as you read this that we are dealing here with an experimental treatment approach. We can, of course, draw from the experiences and formula suggestions made by others that are mentioned here, however when using two highly effective substances simultaneously, there will be an even greater difference between the effects each individual patient will experience than when a single substance is administered. I therefore urge you to become well experienced with using the individual substances singly, and then to inch your way forward taking appropriate care.

2.5.1.1 DMSO and MMS / CDS

With regard to what Jim Humble named MMS (a standardised and activated sodium chlorite solution [$NaClO_2$]), the combination suggestions with DMSO are laid out in Dr Antje Oswald's *The MMS Handbook: Your Health in Your Hands*. If you are keen to experiment, you can mix the MMS solution yourself. Jim Humble has published on the internet precise instructions on how to do this and you should abide strictly by these rules. This ensures that every user across the globe is confident in the knowledge that they are taking exactly the same dose.

Adding the activator causes the effective molecule from this stock solution, namely the chlorine dioxide (ClO_2), to be released. Organic or inorganic acids that are able to give off protons, i.e. hydrogen ions, can be used for this purpose; this includes hydrochloric acid, sulphuric acid or its salts, citric acid, tartaric acid etc. When tartaric acid ($C_4H_6O_6$) is used as an activator, the chemical reaction equation of ClO_2 formation is as follows:

$$5\ NaClO_2 + 4\ C_4H_6O_6 \rightarrow 4\ ClO_2 + 4\ NaC_4H_5O_6 + NaCl + 2\ H_2O$$

It is possible to buy an MMS and activator solution set from a number of internet retailers and pharmacies. As a rule these contain 100ml bottles, which are sufficient for most uses. If you wish to use a different activator, you have the option of buying the MMS solution (22.4%) individually.

Since MMS is used relatively often by people suffering from malignant tumours, I recommend using right-turning lactic acid as an activator. *Lactic acid as activator*

Right turning lactic acid (see Chapter 2.5.4 'DMSO and other (cancer) medications') can be used therapeutically by itself but by using it as an activator you are killing a number of birds with one stone. Firstly, it is an organic acid that can reliably be used to activate the MMS solution and to stabilise it at the same time. Secondly, it is a physiologically active substance that has a number of signalling and detoxifying effects in the human body. Thirdly, as a probiotic, it supports the intestinal flora, which is vitally important for the immune system. You can buy right-turning lactic acid in pharmacies as a 21% preparation. This can then be used in a 1:1 ratio just like the other activators, or add an excess of the (+)-lactic acid (up to 20 drops).

Mixtures of sodium chlorite and lactic acid are more stable, in terms of the decomposition into chloric acid, than the combinations with other organic acids (e.g. citric acid). The 1:1 solution, as so-called 'stabilised chlorine dioxide' or 'Alcide®', also works very well against viruses, fungal nail and warts, and was even used many years ago as a stabiliser against microorganisms.[54] That is another reason why I personally prefer to use right-turning lactic acid as an MMS activator for external use. Lactic acid can be used to produce long-lasting sprays and solutions for the treatment of skin diseases.

External use Jim Humble primarily recommends combining **MMS / CDS with DMSO** for external use to improve absorption through the skin. I also use this method for local, subcutaneous inflammations. Jim Humble recommends working quickly when using this method so that the oxidative power of MMS is not sapped as the reaction with the DMSO begins. As an alternative, he recommends first spraying MMS solution on the skin, then applying the DMSO to that same area of skin. The premature deactivation of these two substances – dimethyl sulfoxide (DMSO) and chlorine dioxide (ClO_2 = the effective molecule in MMS) – is, however, hugely dependent on the concentrations involved. A simple experiment will demonstrate this. A concentrated ClO_2 solution (for example 10 drops MMS and 50 drops of a 10% citric acid), prepared according to Jim Humble's instructions, loses its typical yellow-green chlorine dioxide colour completely within 15 minutes at most when 2ml of DMSO has been added to it.

In contrast, practically no reaction takes place in diluted solutions. Scientific studies show that ClO_2 in diluted, aqueous solutions of DMSO is not reduced or masked in any other way.[55] Noriko Imaizumi and research colleagues at the Niigata College of Pharmacy in Japan did not detect any change in the concentration of ClO_2 after DMSO was added to the pre-acidified (activated) sodium chlorite (MMS). However, they were able to demonstrate that any traces of chlorine present in chlorite or hypochlorite solutions of DMSO are caught very efficiently when water is present. This reaction between DMSO and chlorine, a highly undesirable substance, reduces the chlorine to harmless chloride ions, such as are found in every mineral water. This is a chemical process that requires two electrons. DMSO is oxidised into sulfone, with which we are already familiar.

In other words, it can be useful to add a small quantity of DMSO (less than 1ml) to the MMS drink solution and to take both substances simultaneously. The Japanese scientists talk of a 'small surplus'. For an MMS solution prepared using 3 drops of each of the standard ingredients and topped up with water, it would mean a maximum of 30 milligrams of DMSO – less than 0.03ml. However, that is a theoretical value and these deliberations are only intended to show that mixing DMSO and MMS together in an aqueous solution can be useful: firstly, because of improved tissue penetration of the oxidant ClO_2; and secondly, because any traces of chlorine that may be present disappear. The drink should be taken without delay once the DMSO has been added to it.

Staggered administration is, therefore, not absolutely necessary when taking a combination of DMSO and MMS / CDS internally as a drink. If you do wish to take the MMS / CDS drink solution at a different time from the DMSO, you need not stick to any particular time schedule. As has been explained above, DMSO circulates through the body with favourable effects for many hours after it is taken, which means that you can take the MMS a little earlier or later. Instructions on how to take DMSO as a drink are given in Chapter 2.3. Personally I leave about 30 minutes between taking the two substances.

Pure ClO_2 solutions called CDS (chlorine dioxide solution) are now *Advantages* widely available commercially. These products have a number of advan- *and* tages: they do not contain any of the impurities which can sometimes *disadvantages* find their way into MMS solutions via the sodium chlorite, they are pH *of CDS* neutral, and they can be used immediately from the bottle without needing activation. CDS is better tolerated and safer to use even on sensitive areas such as open wounds, gums and ears. It can even be used (undiluted) directly on insect bites. Due to its mild taste even sensitive people find it possible to increase the dose without problems.

The disadvantage is its short shelf-life in comparison with the standard two-component MMS. Once opened, CDS bottles must be closed again as soon as possible and they must always be stored in a cool, dark place to minimise the loss of efficacy. Significant differences have been established in the chlorine dioxide content of products bought from different retailers, even in freshly delivered bottles – such differences are not really acceptable.

In August 2012 a chlorine dioxide solution in 100ml violet glass bottles came onto the market whose ClO_2 content has been proven, with the aid of photometry, to be reliably stable even after extended storage.

It appears that this is a patented product whose improved stability can be attributed to the special properties of the water – whatever that might mean. Such solutions will probably be very popular with patients because they can be used immediately without activation and the taste is comparatively neutral. Such developments take this substance a huge step towards becoming an user-friendly medication.

Making CDS yourself For me and for other health practitioners who have attended my workshops, preparing a 'home-made' chlorine dioxide solution is the best way to acquire a pure and potent MMS / CDS (infusion-)solution. Personally I only use home-made solutions. To prepare the solution you will need a simple 'ClO_2 generator' with which the gaseous pure substance can be captured in drinking-water or, with the aid of a sterile filter, in the isotonic infusion solution you intend to use. Fresh infusions produced in this way are a particular blessing because they are pH neutral, very effective, and extremely well tolerated. Even my alternative health practitioner students, who are actually perfectly healthy, are always ready to volunteer to demonstrate this procedure because they feel particularly well afterwards.

Jim Humble advises us to be very careful when using MMS infusions because he has repeatedly observed what he assumed were Herxheimer reactions. In complete contrast, however, neither I myself nor other practitioners and self-users I know have ever experienced these reactions. This is despite the fact that our infusions often contain chlorine dioxide released from up to 10 drops(!) of MMS. A colleague and I recently treated an 84-year-old woman suffering from a chronic bacterial infection in this way. The woman felt like a new person after the treatment and proceeded to make us laugh at her anecdotes.

Conclusion

If you produce very pure MMS / CDS infusions they are very well tolerated. I therefore assume that the temporary reactions described in the literature, such as shivering or fever, are caused by impurities (pyrogens) and that they are not 'genuine' Herxheimer reactions. This treatment method should only be used if you have the necessary biochemical and laboratory equipment, which can easily be acquired. With these prerequisites fulfilled, I would personally be very reluctant to give up the CDS infusions because, unlike the drink solutions, they do not cause gastrointestinal complaints even at high doses. The method is so simple that we can only wonder why no one came upon the idea much earlier. We teach and practise this method at our workshops.

What is the dosage or potency relationship between the new CDS and *CDS doses* the classic MMS solutions? According to the manufacturers, CDS contains a maximum of 0.3% ClO_2 – that is 3 grams in a litre of water (although as I stated above, it is uncertain how accurate this figure is in many cases). By this measure, one millilitre of such a solution would contain 3mg of chlorine dioxide. Assuming a standard drop volume of 0.05ml, expect a maximum of 0.15mg ClO_2 per drop of CDS.

According to stoichiometric calculations, a standard MMS solution (22.4% $NaClO_2$) contains, in theory, a maximum of about 6.5mg of ClO_2 per drop. This is when you calculate ClO_2 formation using the chemical equation and assume that the reaction process proceeds optimally. That would suggest that MMS is about 40 times stronger than CDS. So if the content information on the 0.3% CDS bottle was accurate, and if the standard MMS solution reacts fully into ClO_2, a 2ml (= 40 drops) dose of CDS is equal to one drop of MMS.

So much for the theory. We know from various photometric laboratory experiments that the activation reaction of the aqueous sodium chlorite standard solution (MMS) with the acid added in an open glass yields a suboptimal quantity of ClO_2.

What does that mean exactly? We are accustomed to putting a certain number of drops of the usual 22.4% sodium chlorite solution into

a glass and adding the 'appropriate' number of drops of a suitable activator. This activator is an acid that changes the pH value of the MMS
drops from being very alkaline to being acidic. The chemical formation
reaction of the actual effective substance chlorine dioxide then begins
once a pH value of less than 7 is reached. At room temperature chlorine
dioxide is gaseous and immediately begins to escape into the air. That is
apparent from the small gas bubbles that form in the mixture. Fill the
glass with water. This greatly dilutes the solution and the activation reaction, which is not completely finished after a period of a few seconds,
slows down considerably. At the same time the ClO_2 that has already
been produced and is still being dissolved in the mixture is 'bound' to
the added water. At 4 °C, the solubility of chlorine dioxide in water is
20 parts per 1 part water. That would be about 20ml of gaseous ClO_2
(approx. 50mg) in 1ml of water. Solubility is proportionately less at room
temperature. This ready-to-drink MMS solution is a yellow-green colour
because of the ClO_2 it contains. The two stock solutions (sodium chlorite and the activator) are almost colourless. The light absorption of col-
oured solutions can be tested if you know the wavelength that is 'swallowed' by the substance; this is called the maximum absorption. For
ClO_2 this is at a light wavelength of 360nm (nanometre), which is within
the ultraviolet spectral range. The concentration of the absorbing substance in the water can be inferred if you use a photometer to measure
the reduction in the radiated wavelength behind the glass container (cu-
vette) in which the solution is stored.

For example, this test reveals that a drink made by adding 6 drops of
a 50% tartaric acid solution to 6 drops of MMS and waiting 30 seconds
before adding 250ml of water has a ClO_2 content of 4.8mg (measurement reading: 19mg per litre). That is considerably less than the 6.5mg
ClO_2 per drop of MMS that you would expect in theory. What is the explanation for this? Firstly, some of the ClO_2 produced escapes into the
air before the water is added. That is why we can smell it in the room.
Secondly, the reaction whereby sodium chlorite changes to chlorine
dioxide is not complete at the moment the water is added. The drink
solutions are therefore subject to a certain amount of 'post-ripening'. But
at the same time, because the substance continues to escape from the
water and to break down because of the light, the photometer cannot
detect any increase in concentration worth speaking of. There is therefore a dilemma because a longer activation period would lead to an even
greater loss of gas.

A number of different preparation methods (including the Gefeu Method, for example) that aim to bypass these problems are listed in Dr Antje Oswald's *The MMS Handbook: Your Health in Your Hands*.

Moreover, chemical reactions conducted in test tubes, even under optimal conditions, almost never achieve a 100% yield. According to the equation reaction, 5 parts sodium chlorite would, in theory, yield 4 parts chlorine dioxide. However, as the photometric measurements have shown, the drop mixture method does not yield anything of the sort. So in contrast to defined, standardised medication solutions that have reliable indications of the percentage contained within (e.g. 3% H_2O_2 solutions), there are various 'losses' and other influencing factors to consider when using the normal MMS solution.

Photometric testing has also shown that 6 drops of stabilised CDS (labelled as being <0.3%) in 250ml of water yields 5.7mg ClO_2 per litre. So you would need to multiply this by 3.3 to equal the above measurement of 19mg/l for 6 drops of MMS activated using the standard method.

Conclusion

For dose purposes, the ratio between (at best) a 0.3% CDS and the standard MMS solution would be around 3.5 to 1.

3 to 4 drops CDS = 1 drop MMS

The practical experience of my patients and other practitioners continues to be inconsistent in this regard. However, I often hear that patients intuitively feel CDS to be less effective. That would probably be down to the patient taking an incorrect / too low a dose, or to the potency of the solution being too weak. We know that the 'home-made' CDS described above has long proven itself to be a highly effective medication in practical application.

The photometric measurements of the various chlorine dioxide solutions currently available have shown that the 0.3% ClO_2 content declared on the packaging is not always accurate. It is to be hoped that manufacturers of such solutions adopt standardised quality criteria. It would be a shame if the admirable innovation of ready-to-use chlorine dioxide solution, and the success achieved through its use, was tarnished simply because some amateurs attempt to jump onto the (sales) bandwagon selling goods of insufficient concentration. After all, as an end user, you want reliable products or substances and it is worth making the effort to find them.

The medical literature does not provide uniform instructions on how to prepare combinations of DMSO and MMS 2, a diluted aqueous calcium hypochlorite solution $(Ca(ClO)_2)$ which yields hypochlorous acid as the active compound. However, users are constantly posting relevant experiences and methods on internet forums. With some practice, self-observation, and on your own responsibility, you should be able to find your way with these substances too.

Hypochlorite solutions have been and continue to be used in medicine to disinfect wounds because they are such effective oxidants. This substance is commonly used to rinse an open tooth socket as part of root canal treatment. However, in such cases solutions containing relatively high concentrations of about 5% are used. Significantly lower concentrations of hypochlorite are used for the therapeutic applications outlined here. When using MMS 2, Jim Humble states that capsules should be filled with 400 milligrams of calcium hypochlorite (about 70% quality). It is recommended that you drink 3 glasses of water with one of these capsules. That is a total of 0.6 to 0.9 litres, depending on the glass. Even if we base the calculation on only 0.5 litres, that would still only give a concentration of 0.08% for one 400mg capsule. Maximum concentrations of 0.5% are recommended for external application to rinse wounds, and a maximum of 0.005% for therapeutic baths to treat atopic eczema (atopic dermatitis).

Based on extensive experience of using MMS / CDS, we can calculate a reasonable concentration for calcium hypochlorite solutions as follows.

MMS 2   Jim Humble defines an MMS solution as a 28% mixture of a 80% sodium chlorite solution and water. Accordingly, 100ml of such a solution contains 22.4 grams of pure $NaClO_2$. Let us assume we want to imitate a dose of 5 drops of MMS 1. Generally speaking, 5 drops corresponds to one quarter of a millilitre (50μl per drop). If 100ml of the standard solution contains 22.4 grams of sodium chlorite, then 0.25ml contains 0.056 grams or 56 milligrams. Calcium hypochlorite is a completely different chemical compound that has a different molecular weight from sodium chlorite and this must be accounted for in the calculation. The molecular weight of $NaClO_2$ is $M = 90.4$ gram per mole, the molecular weight of $Ca(ClO)_2$ is M = 143g per mole. A simple calculation reveals that 56mg of MMS 1 is equivalent to 88.6mg of MMS 2. However, this is true only for the pure substance. Since the commonly available product is 70% calcium hypochlorite (the remainder is mainly calcium hydroxide), we need to divide this quantity by 0.7, giving us 126.6mg. That would be the quantity of MMS 2 from which we could expect a similar oxidative effect as we would obtain from 5 drops of MMS 1. This calculation is overly simplified because calcium hypochlorite mixed in a water solution yields two hypochlorous acid molecules, as this formula states:

$$Ca(ClO)_2 + 2\,H_2O \rightarrow 2\,HOCl + 2\,OH^- + Ca^{2+}$$

These molecules, in turn, can only be approximately compared with a ClO_2 molecule, which can transfer two oxygen atoms or a total of five electrons. Despite that, the approximate figure of 125mg of calcium hypochlorite that the calculation gives us is a useful guiding value. Since the calculation was originally based on 5 drops of MMS, we can estimate that 25mg of MMS 2 powder corresponds roughly to one drop of MMS in terms of oxidative effect. Based on these figures, Dr Antje Oswald in her book *The MMS Handbook: Your Health in Your Hands* recommends starting with a dose of 50mg of MMS 2 powder when you are making initial tolerance tests on your own responsibility. That would be the equivalent of taking a starting dose of 2 drops of MMS.

DMSO and MMS 2

Combining DMSO and a diluted HOCl solution has proven useful because, as mentioned above, pure hypochlorite solutions can contain traces of elemental chlorine. Chlorine is a toxic substance, as you probably know from reports on the criticisms made of public swimming pools (which are only disinfected using chlorine dioxide, i.e. MMS / CDS, in 'rich' countries – a group to which Germany clearly does not belong according to this definition). However, when DMSO is added, any traces of chlorine that may be present are masked and reduced to chloride ions. In such cases the DMSO not only improves the ability of the dissolved hypochlorite to penetrate tissue, it also makes the solution even safer for external and internal use. However, hypochlorous acid (HOCl) in the low pH range can oxidise DMSO, even in diluted solutions. Directly mixing DMSO and diluted calcium chlorite solutions is therefore only advised when the pH value does not fall too far under 7 or when the solution is diluted strongly. Only then is there no detectable reaction between DMSO and HOCl.

Intake method   Use the staggered intake method (as described in the previous section for MMS and DMSO) when combining larger quantities of DMSO and MMS 2 for internal use. First take the desired quantities of calcium hypochlorite capsules, following Jim Humble's recommendations. You must drink a large amount of water – two glasses beforehand and one glass afterwards. The MMS 2 capsules can be easily opened which means that you can, for example, take a quarter of the calcium hypochlorite contained if you carefully pour out ¾ of the content and then close the capsule again. Warning: the powder is very aggressive in its pure form. It is best to trickle it directly into a large quantity of water so that you can dispose of this diluted solution without burning the skin with the powder. Then take the DMSO as usual, for example 3.5ml dissolved in a 300ml drink.

You can also do this in reverse. First take the diluted DMSO and then take the MMS 2 capsule with plenty of water. That may strike you as being an extremely large quantity of liquid to take. After all, 4 glasses add up to 1.2 litres. The total volume can be reduced somewhat if you mix the DMSO into the first glass of water you drink before taking the MMS 2 capsule or that you drink after taking the capsule. This would also help to mask any chlorine that may be contained, as explained above. There is also the option of administering DMSO in parallel as an infusion if drinking so much water gets too much for you. The potential advantage of parallel DMSO and hypochlorous acid administration should be obvious: DMSO is used to make certain that the hypochlorous acid penetrates the tissue more deeply and more quickly, and is thereby available to support immune defence processes.

When using stronger concentrations of aqueous hypochlorite solutions (MMS 2 in water e.g. 0.5% to 1%) externally in combination with DMSO, the substances are administered in the same order as is the case for DMSO and MMS / CDS. The oxidative solution (in this case calcium hypochlorite in water) is applied first, followed by the DMSO solution. This is because when a concentrated mixture of the oxidative hypochlorous acid (HOCl) and DMSO is left to stand for too long, the HOCl oxidises the DMSO into MSM. That saps the hypochlorous acid's power before it can be put to use. This should be avoided in order to ensure that you achieve the full effect.

2.5.1.2 DMSO and hydrogen peroxide

Hydrogen peroxide (H_2O_2 or 'superoxide') is also an oxidative substance. It has long been and still is in use as an industrial bleach and as a medical disinfectant. You are probably also familiar with its use as a hair dye and as a teeth whitener. Until the 1980s it was commonly found in home medicine kits and in doctors' surgeries, where it was used to disinfect wounds (e.g. 1.5% solutions). To disinfect wounds? But that would seem to suggest that it kills microorganisms and parasites!

Hydrogen peroxide has suffered a fate similar to that of the other substances we have already looked at. Even though it was used medicinally with great success many years ago, the pharmaceutical lobby has since turned its back on it because it is of little commercial interest. That is the reason why no clinical trials have been conducted on it. However, holistic doctors and alternative practitioners have documented a wide range of amazing effects and gathered numerous interesting users' reports.[56,57] With regard to therapeutic use, aqueous H_2O_2 solution has the following distinctive features that set it apart from MMS and MMS 2. Firstly, the substance is odourless and the taste is neutral (depending on concentration). Secondly, oxygen concentrations in the blood and / or the tissue are noticeably higher soon after it is taken internally. This effect, examined later in more detail, occurs because the body has a substantial wealth of enzymes that can transform H_2O_2 quickly into oxygen and water.

Distinctive features of hydrogen peroxide

If you cast your mind back, you will remember that hydrogen peroxide is produced by our body's own defence cells and that the body must have effective mechanisms with which to regulate such oxidative substances. Hydrogen peroxide has two different biochemical decomposition reactions which run in parallel. In one case (1) it leads to the formation of oxygen atoms that have an oxidative effect, killing off microorganisms. In the second case (2), influenced by specific enzymes, 'normal', molecular oxygen is formed, which helps to improve tissue supply. In both cases the only by-product is water (H_2O).

$$1. \quad H_2O_2 \quad \rightarrow \quad [O] + H_2O$$
$$2. \quad 2\,H_2O_2 \quad \rightarrow \quad O_2 + 2\,H_2O$$

As indicated by the standard potentials shown in Table 2, the oxidative power of H_2O_2 is greater than that of MMS / CDS and MMS 2. Like CDS, hydrogen peroxide does not need to be activated by adding acid (low pH value) in order to become reactive. There is therefore no reason why you cannot prepare a solution of this superoxide at a pH of 7 or slightly below so that you are within range of normal blood pH values. In that case the oxidation potential of H_2O_2 decreases to 1.4V, i.e. it becomes milder and the drink solution becomes easier to tolerate. The pH values of aqueous solutions can be raised (made more alkaline) by adding small quantities of sodium bicarbonate.

You can buy hydrogen peroxide solutions in specified concentrations (e.g. 3%) in pharmacies. Laboratory and aquarium suppliers sell stabilised concentrations of 30 to 35% H_2O_2 in 1-litre bottles, which can then be appropriately diluted for external use. Example: use a pipette or syringe to draw 1ml of a 30% solution and top that up to 10ml with water, giving you a 3% hydrogen peroxide solution. If you take 8.6ml of a 35% source solution and top that up with water to 100ml, this will also provide you with a 3% solution.

> **Caution**
>
> The concentrated 30 or 35% hydrogen peroxide solution is extremely corrosive! It must not come into contact with the skin or eyes and should not be swallowed. When handling this substance always wear safety clothing: suitable gloves, lab coat and **protective glasses**. Bottles must always be labelled clearly, in accordance with regulations. Keep out of the reach of children. Observe all the instructions on the relevant safety leaflet. Particular care should be taken to ensure that contact with metal is avoided.

As with the other substances discussed, you should pay close attention to the quality of the hydrogen peroxide you buy. If at all possible always buy the pharmaceutical grade (Ph. Eur.) hydrogen peroxide, otherwise it may contain dubious stabilisers. Depending on the application you have in mind you should use purified water to dilute; sterile, isotonic saline solution is also suitable.

H_2O_2 *doses* What dose of H_2O_2 is best? Using the oxidation power of MMS as a point of orientation, and taking the MMS dose guidelines as a basis, it is necessary to bear in mind that the molecular weight of hydrogen peroxide (34 gram per mole) is much lower than that of chlorine dioxide (67.5 gram per mole). This means that you would only need to use approximately half the quantity of hydrogen peroxide in comparison with the quantity of MMS. According to photometric measurements, 1 drop of MMS (= 0.05ml) produces about 0.4mg ClO_2 in the drink solution; that is the equivalent of about 0.2mg of H_2O_2. If a 3% solution is used, this 0.2mg of H_2O_2 would be contained in 0.007ml, i.e. about one-seventh of a drop. The calculation is as follows:

$$100 \text{ ml } 3\% \text{ } H_2O_2 \text{ solution} \cong 3000 \text{ milligrams } H_2O_2$$
$$x \text{ ml} \cong 0.2 \text{ milligrams } H_2O_2$$
$$\rightarrow x = 0{,}007 \text{ ml}$$

This figure must be doubled because the effective component of activated MMS solution (chlorine dioxide) can transfer two oxygen atoms, while H_2O_2 can only transfer one.

In theory therefore, ¼ drop of a 3% H_2O_2 solution would have roughly the same oxidative power as one drop of MMS solution. In reverse, the oxidative power of 1 drop of this hydrogen peroxide solution would be similar to that of 4 drops of MMS.

Armed with this information you can use hydrogen peroxide in various ways, as you are accustomed to doing with MMS. In his book, Josef Pies[56] describes a number of amazing methods and applications that medical lay people can use to treat humans, animals and plants. Among them is a method for a spray application of H_2O_2 together with DMSO, which helps to improve absorption. According to Pies, hydrogen peroxide infusion treatments (which should only be carried out by doctors and alternative health practitioners) have been successfully used to treat a number of serious illnesses, including arthritis, candida, MS, varicose veins, chronic fatigue syndrome, rheumatism and cancer.

Combining H_2O_2 and DMSO is of particular interest with regard to cancer. Cancer cells have two particular characteristics that distinguish them from healthy or 'normal' cells. Firstly, their metabolic processes switch to utilising glucose anaerobically (without oxygen). That means that they carry out relatively ineffective and wasteful fermentation processes in the cell plasma, rather than optimised oxidation processes within the mitochondria (the Warburg hypothesis, formulated by Otto Warburg (1883–1970), Nobel Prize for Medicine / Physiology 1931). Mitochondria are parts of the cell (organelles) that are often called 'power stations' because they produce energy from glucose and oxygen

Understanding cancer

through a process called cell respiration. Carbon dioxide is the 'only' by-product of this process. Secondly, when the mitochondria are closed down, it leads to the loss of apoptosis capability. Apoptosis is the process of programmed cell death. Cells usually know when something within them is not right, or when something is moving away from the expected course. When this happens they bring about their own demise. The reactive oxygen species (e.g. peroxides) belong to the group of messenger substances that initiate this process. This is nature's mechanism to prevent the further expansion of degenerate cells. Based on this knowledge, a number of medical practitioners believe that cancer is ultimately caused by oxygen deficiency in the tissue.

Looked at from another perspective, cancer cells appear not to like it when the concentration of oxygen in their surroundings or in the cells themselves rises. This is exactly what can be achieved through the administration of H_2O_2. Adding DMSO causes hydrogen peroxide to be transported even more effectively to the cells.

Superoxide infusions   Knowing this, if we look again at the research carried out by Finney and his colleagues at the Medical Faculty of Dallas University[43] we can understand the interrelationships more clearly. The scientists analysed the heart muscle performance of pigs that had been treated with an infusion of 0.06% H_2O_2 and 10% DMSO in an electrolyte solution. The researchers attributed the positive results to the fact that this combination of substances is a particularly effective way of improving the oxygen supply to the (muscle) tissue because the DMSO transports the H_2O_2 into the thick heart muscle. The results were far less impressive when infusions containing only one of the two substances, DMSO or hydrogen peroxide, were administered.

Assuming that these were 1-litre infusion bottles, the solution would contain 0.6 grams of H_2O_2 and 100g of DMSO, and 0.6 grams of hydrogen peroxide is equivalent to about 20 millilitres of the standard 3% solution (density variations disregarded). That is about 400 drops! The pigs were able to tolerate these infusions but such quantities are far beyond the quantities of oxidants that we have experience of administering to humans. According to Ed McCabe© a 500ml isotonic infusion containing a maximum of 5ml of 3% hydrogen peroxide is used to treat adult patients. This method has a particularly beneficial effect on the skin, making it appear more youthful.

Since hydrogen peroxide is a much stronger oxidant than MMS, the pH value should be checked after adding and mixing the DMSO. H_2O_2

is more stable in the acidic range (pH value < 7) than in the alkaline range. Sodium bicarbonate ($NaHCO_3$) can be used to adjust the pH value of the solution upwards, while magnesium chloride ($MgCl_2$) can be used to adjust the pH value downwards. By doing so you can avoid prematurely losing the oxidative power of the hydrogen peroxide through its reaction with DMSO. Electrolyte infusions as used by Finney when preparing the H_2O_2 / DMSO combinations are fine because the various salts contained within work as pH buffers.

The basic guidelines set out in Chapter 2.4 'Administration by injection' should be observed when preparing combination infusions of DMSO and hydrogen peroxide. The same suggested doses can be followed when the substances are used individually or in combination with other substances. You should always carry out the relevant tolerance tests beforehand.

Infusion solution combinations of oxidative substances and DMSO should only be prepared shortly before use, and should be kept in darkness under a towel while you are administering them. The drop rate must be set at an appropriately slow speed to avoid causing irritation to the veins, and the patient should be under constant observation. It should be clear that this kind of high-potency treatment must only be carried out by experienced therapists (doctors and alternative health practitioners) who are legally authorised to do so. When administering a 500ml isotonic saline solution infusion, start with 0.1g DMSO per kilogram of body weight and 10 drops of a 3% hydrogen peroxide solution. This treatment can be given every other day at the most. If this is tolerated well, the quantity can be doubled to 0.2g DMSO/kg body weight and 20 drops H_2O_2 (1ml). It is important to maintain the aseptic chain and to filter all the substances before they are administered into the sterile infusion.

To summarise: we know that when DMSO and hydrogen peroxide are combined, each substance complements and reinforces the therapeutic effect of the other. While H_2O_2 predominantly works to fight microorganisms and to improve oxygen supply to the tissue, DMSO improves the availability of hydrogen peroxide. DMSO also improves blood circulation, inhibits inflammation, and works as a free radical scavenger. Combined use improves the treatment results in practically all the diseases that have so far been treated by the two substances singly.

2.5.2 DMSO and procaine

Procaine is a local anaesthetic. It was first synthesised by the German chemist Alfred Einhorn in Munich at the beginning of the twentieth century and was introduced onto the market in 1905 by the Höchst pharmaceutical company under the name Novocaine®. Previous to that, cocaine had been commonly used as a local anaesthetic and it had been Einhorn's intention to find a substance that was better tolerated.

Discovery   Unrelated to the substance's use as an anaesthetic in dentistry and medicine, in 1925 the two physicians Ferdinand and Walter Huneke discovered procaine's many therapeutic properties. They subsequently developed what they termed neural therapy and interference field therapy, where procaine solutions are used on potential interference fields such as scars or inflamed sinuses. Due to the postulated 'action at a distance', chronic illnesses caused by these interference fields can be cured. The story of the Huneke brothers and the development of their medical method is an exciting chapter in the history of medicine which I highly recommend you read.

Effects   Procaine, both as a medicine and in terms of its neural therapy application, is of great interest as a combination substance with DMSO. Scientific testing has shown that procaine inhibits the nervous conduction of the neuron axons by blocking the ion channels in the cell membranes.[59] Because pain signals are conducted 'electrically' along the nerve fibre with the aid of rapid changes in voltage, the inhibition of the ion migration of sodium ions (and others) along these channels leads to a reversible impairment of function and therefore to numbness and the anaesthetisation of the affected tissue. This can 'reset' the nerve function in a very particular way. This is one effect (among others) that the Huneke brothers attribute to the amazing results brought about by the 'phenomenon of seconds' in a successful neural therapy treatment.

Along with the anaesthetic effect, procaine exhibits further characteristics typical for this class of medications. It has a spasmolytic effect, meaning that it relieves cramping in the smooth muscle tissue such as is found in the blood vessels, the gastrointestinal tract, the biliary tract and in the urinary passage. It has a sympatholytic effect in that it temporarily inhibits the sympathetic part of the involuntary nervous system. This can help improve blood circulation to the arms and legs. Procaine also has an antihistamine effect (it inhibits allergic reactions) and an antiarrhythmic effect (it regulates heart rhythm disturbances).

Procaine's superior status when compared with other local anaes-thetics is based on its unique combination of other biologically signi-ficant effects. The most important of these are the vasodilatory effect that even improves circulation in the fine capillaries (= improves per-fusion) and its anti-inflammatory, antioxidant and oxygen-conserving characteristics.

Due to the inhibiting effect it has on the monoamine oxidase (MAO), a group of enzymes that break down serotonin and dopamine, procaine can even have a regulating effect on neurotransmitter balance, thereby resolving psychogenic symptoms.

To summarise: procaine is known to be extremely useful not only as part of the neural therapy approach described above, but also in the systemic treatment of severe chronic inflammations and pain syn-dromes. It is also recognised today as an effective substance by holisti-cally-minded conventional doctors.

The only significant material disadvantage of procaine is its poor dis-tribution performance in body tissue. That is the reason why it has been widely replaced by other substances in dentistry and medicine. Bells must already be ringing at the mention of the word 'distribution' without the necessity of reminding readers of DMSO's impressive performance as a transporter of other substances. If we value the pharmacological ef-fects of procaine, and if its only drawback lies in difficulties distributing the substance in the tissue, then we can easily and naturally solve the problem by combining procaine with DMSO. *DMSO offsets disadvantage*

Another aspect of the pharmacological properties of procaine that deserves consideration is the fact that this molecule can only pass through cell walls in an uncharged state, as a neutral particle, before then unleashing its effect on the aforementioned ion channels 'from the inside'. The presence of acids that are able to give off hydrogen ions, or more generally a low pH value, leads to a hydrogen ion coupling with the nitrogen atom (N) in the procaine, which changes the procaine itself into an ion, i.e. a charged particle. Inflamed tissue usually has a low pH value. From the perspective of neural therapy, such inflammations ben-efit in particular from procaine administration. Depending on temper-ature and electrolyte concentration, the pK_a value of procaine (= acidity constant) is about 8 to 9,[60] meaning that even at a neutral pH value of 7.0, 99% of the procaine molecules are present in the form of charged procaineH$^+$ cations. *Procaine needs a high pH value*

The mathematical equation for acid–alkaline reaction equilibrium reveals that around 90% of the free, uncharged procaine is available if the pH value lies at around 1 above the pK_a value – so between 9 and 10.

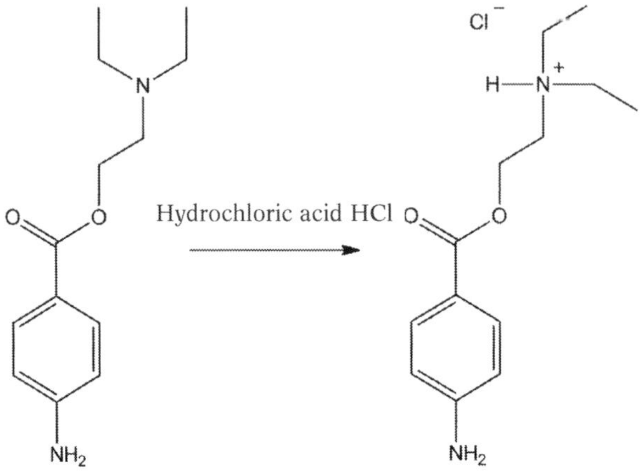

Figure 35: Procaine is converted by an acid (in this case hydrochloric acid, HCl) into a charged particle (cation).

The ionic form of procaine shown here, the charged particle known as procaine hydrochloride, is the normal form of the medicine available commercially. The ampules contain 10% hydrochloric acid to lower the pH value for this purpose. After being administered, the procaine hydrochloride has to be first (partially) converted back to an uncharged state by an appropriately alkaline pH value > 8, so that the desired effects can take place optimally within the cells.

That means that the infiltrative treatment of a chronically inflamed scar using procaine alone may be unsuccessful because the substance cannot flow into the affected nerve cells. How can this problem be solved? Think back to figure 8 in Chapter 1. Cations (positively charged particles) such as the procaine cation depicted here are transported particularly well by DMSO through biological membranes. Combining procaine and DMSO therefore makes particularly good sense because the latter, as we have already learned, has an anti-inflammatory effect of its own and can build a molecular 'shell' around the procaine. As a result, the procaine, aided by its 'carrier', arrives in the cells practically without obstruction. Alternatively-minded doctors also like to administer procaine by mixing it with sodium bicarbonate in appropriate concentrations. The sodium bicarbonate leads to a local alkalisation of the tissue, elevating the pH value, which means that more uncharged procaine molecules can penetrate the cell membranes. This also leads to improved / prolonged effect.[61]

Procaine is an ester of the para-aminobenzoic acid (PABA). This compound is important in a biological sense as a building block in folic acid synthesis in the (intestinal) bacteria. PABA is used as an ingredient in sunscreens because it absorbs UV light, and it is also used as a nutritional supplement (vitamin B10). I mention this because I am often asked whether a synthetically produced substance, in this case procaine, is acceptable as an alternative therapy. Procaine is broken down in the tissue or in the blood by an enzyme (pseudocholinesterase) into PABA and diethylaminoethanol (DEAE, which also has a vasodilatory effect). This enzyme, an abundance of which is present in our bodies, is usually required to convert the neurotransmitter (messenger of the nerve cells) acetylcholine.

Despite that, it should be remembered that allergic reactions to procaine can occur in rare cases. To eliminate this risk every user should carry out an individual tolerance test before using procaine, as is done before using DMSO. Do this by inducing a small wheal on the lower arm using the widely available 0.5 to 2% procaine solution. The wheal should disappear within 20 minutes leaving no sign of irritation. The length of time can, however, vary greatly from individual to individual.

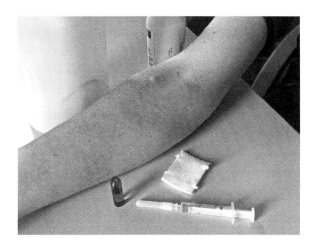

Figure 36: Wheal on the skin of the lower arm with 1% procaine

The article by Reuter and Oettmeier,[61] among others, reports that the widely held opinion regarding the danger of allergic reactions to procaine must now be reconsidered. It was long believed that para-compounds (such as PABA) generally caused such symptoms. Today, however, procaine is regarded and valued as a very safe substance. The number of (neural therapy) treatments administered is enormous, and the trend is increasing.

Method   If you passed the wheal test, you can use the DMSO–procaine combinations. The simplest method is to mix a 2ml solution from a standard procaine vial (0.5 to 2%) with an equal amount of DMSO. This yields a 50% DMSO solution containing 10 to 40mg of procaine hydrochloride. Was that too quick? Here are the calculations:

> 1 vial of a 1% procaine solution contains 2ml water
> → 1% of 2000mg = 20mg procaine

> 2ml aqueous procaine solution + 2ml DMSO
> → 50% aqueous DMSO solution

To obtain a higher concentration of DMSO, add (for example) 3ml DMSO to the 2ml procaine solution. This yields a 60% DMSO solution.

You can now apply this mixture externally directly onto painful inflammations, irritated scars, myogelosis etc. DMSO deploys its own beneficial effects locally, as well as transporting the procaine into deeper skin and tissue layers.

If you are authorised to do so, observing the relevant hygiene rules (see Chapter 2.4), you can administer this as an intra- and subcutaneous or intramuscular treatment. A practical way in which to do so is to first draw up 2ml of the procaine solution into a 5ml syringe and then, after fitting a suitable sterile syringe filter, draw up the desired quantity of DMSO (e.g. 1ml).

To administer a high-dose DMSO–procaine infusion, start by following the instructions in Chapter 2.4. Once you have added the DMSO to the infusion solution, all the while complying with the strict hygiene and sterilisation rules, add the necessary quantity of procaine solution. You can also add sodium bicarbonate solution (basic salts). This raises the pH value of the infusion solution, creating favourable conditions for the procaine to unleash its full effect in the body tissue.

Example: take a 500ml infusion bottle containing isotonic saline solution and top this up with the above quantities of DMSO (0.1 to 0.5g/kg body weight), 0.1 to 0.5g procaine as a 2% solution, and 10 to 120ml of standard 8.4% $NaHCO_3$ solution. If you want to start cautiously, when treating a patient weighing 70kg the formula is as follows:

500ml isotonic NaCl solution
7ml DMSO (0.11g per kg body weight)
5ml 2% procaine solution (= 100mg procaine)
50ml 8.4% $NaHCO_3$ solution

One common way in which these infusions are applied is as a series of daily administrations lasting for one to two weeks. They are typically used to improve and accelerate healing following operations (and also used beforehand), pain syndromes following operations on the spine, neuralgias, dystrophies (e.g. Sudeck's atrophy), rheumatism, chronic inflammatory bowel diseases, pancreatic inflammations, withdrawal syndrome, circulation problems, strokes / heart attacks etc. As you can see, this represents a valuable enrichment of the therapeutic repertoire when it comes to treating some serious illnesses and severe pain. However, it is vital that you practice and study this application and have mastered its use. The therapist and patient are, of course, acting on their own responsibility here. If you, as a patient, are suffering from one of these severe illnesses and believe that the substance combinations described here could alleviate your symptoms or cure you completely, then you should take care to find an experienced therapist. You could start by trying out the methods and combinations 'for domestic use' that do not require the use of an injection needle. You will then acquire a feel for the way in which DMSO–procaine combinations affect you.

Fields of application

2.5.3 DMSO and haematoxylin

Haematoxylin is a 'colourless substance extracted from logwood (haematoxylum campechianum) that is easily oxidised in air (or by oxidisers) to become haematein, a red dye'.[62] Haematoxylin and haematein solutions have been used in the field of histology to dye microscopic tissue samples for over 150 years. They have also been used for medicinal purposes, e.g. as an astringent and an anti-inflammatory treatment, for a long while. Haematoxylin is also used as a special titration method for plant compounds.

The molecular structure reveals that this natural plant dye contains five hydroxyl groups (OH-). These oxygenated structural parts generally make a substance readily water-soluble, as is the case with sugar molecules, for example. However, the haematoxylin particles also contain what is known as nonpolar structural parts that reduce this solubility. We will be returning to these characteristics shortly.

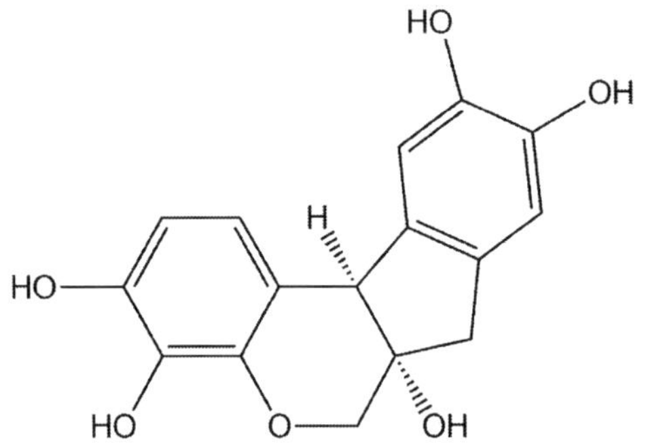

Figure 37: Molecule diagram of the plant dye haematoxylin

Application as a cancer treatment The remarkable thing about this dye is that it principally attaches to acidic cell structures, which it then marks. We can also use this laboratory procedure 'in vivo', i.e. we can mark acidic tissue directly in the body. This is done using a combination of haematoxylin with DMSO. Dr Morton Walker calls this procedure 'The DMSO–Cancer Connection'.[19] You can immediately draw the conclusion that DMSO and haematoxylin mixtures can be implemented in the battle against cancer. Dr Morton refers to the work of Dr Eli Jordon Tucker in the 1960s and 1970s, work which has been ignored by the medical cancer establishment to this day.[63]

Morton Walker describes the case of a 56-year-old Exxon Oil manager who was suffering from advanced stage colorectal cancer. The diagnosis was made in April 1974 after the patient had noticed bleeding from the bowel. He refused conventional chemotherapy treatment and turned to Dr Tucker who treated him with DMSO–haematoxylin infusions. Eighteen months later the man was in such good health that he was regarded as having been cured. The general tumour marker CEA was no longer detectable.

In 1978, after Dr Tucker had published work describing a number of such cases, the FDA became interested in this approach to cancer treatment. However, after receiving a request for more study results, nothing happened. Dr Morton suspects that the matter was, once again, left to peter out for political and commercial reasons.

It was a chance discovery that led Dr Tucker to the DMSO–haematoxylin mixture. He was a highly esteemed physician who had received many awards and he was a leading researcher who had made advancements in bone tissue transplant methods. He used calf bones from a nearby abattoir in his experiments. Out of curiosity and in the search for 'cancer antibodies', in the early 1960s he began to research the blood of cattle that had clearly suffered from cancer before being slaughtered. He then injected the isolated gamma globulins into mice and rats that suffered from cancer. He spent a long time searching for the perfect dye so that he would be able to observe the effects in the animal tissue on a microscopic level. Haematoxylin had the desired characteristic of displaying the tumorous cells in a typical colour. However, it has very poor solubility, which led Tucker to use liquid DMSO. Haematoxylin is very soluble in DMSO and DMSO does not cause any change in the dye. When combined with DMSO, haematoxylin is channelled directly into the tumour cells. It is disseminated there and fastens itself in a chemically stable way onto cell structures that are multi-charged, for example onto the DNA in the cell nucleus. Because of the low pH in this environment, these structures appear under the microscope in violet-blue. *The history of its discovery*

Astonishingly, in experiments on healthy dogs Tucker discovered that a mixture of 25g of haematoxylin and 75ml of DMSO, given as an infusion in electrolyte solution, was tolerated extremely well. The mixture was also tolerated significantly better by rats than was the individual substance. He thereupon tried these infusion solutions on animals suffering from cancer. One of the animals he treated was a friend's dog. The dog had a large-cell malignant lymphoma ('lymph node cancer') and had multiple tumours throughout its body. The swelling in the throat had very nearly led to the dog suffocating. The owner asked Dr Tucker whether he could help the dog in some way, or whether the dog should be put down. After daily administration of the DMSO–haematoxylin infusion mixture for two weeks all the tumours had disappeared and after a thorough examination the dog was pronounced cured. Once recovered and recuperated he sadly ate a large piece of poisoned meat and died. As a result Tucker had an unusual opportunity to examine tissue samples under the microscope. He did *Treating dogs* not find a single recognisable tumour cell, only the so-called 'ghost cells', remnants of the dead cancer cells.

A number of further experiments have shown that various kinds of malignant tumours respond differently to this treatment, not all of them positively. However, Tucker continued his research in a systematic and structured manner and eventually developed a standard dose for use in humans and began to treat cancer patients. Dr Morton Walker has published the treatment protocol and results of 37 patients from the early *Systemic* years of the research (pp. 186–93).[19] In those days treatment results *application* were very much dependent on the type of cancer under observation. The relevant administration method (infusion, drink solution, spray) is based on the location of the tumour and other factors.

Unfortunately, Dr Tucker did not publish any further results regarding the treatments administered after 1968 because he feared the consequences for his standing within the profession. Nevertheless, Walker describes other cases that indicate that there is a good chance of a cure when this method is used to treat malignant lymphomas in particular. Giant-cell tumours (thighbone), skin melanomas and cervical cancers were also successfully treated. Dr Tucker was very aggrieved that a number of colleagues criticised or even threatened him; later he only treated severely ill individuals who turned to him. He took little or no money for treatments, and he did not wish to attract any publicity to his anti-cancer treatment. We are indebted to Morton Walker for the information we have today after Eli Jordan Tucker died shortly before his book was published.

Mode You will now be asking yourself how haematoxylin actually works. Why *of action* does the administration of an organic, biological dye lead to the demise of cancer cells?

Morton Walker[19] reports on research work carried out by Thomas D. Rogers at the North Texas State University. Rogers, a PhD graduate, carried out light and electron microscope analysis on the affected tissue of mice suffering from lymph node cancer, under the supervision of Dr Vernon Scholes. Two important findings were made following the administration of a DMSO–haematoxylin mixture by means of an intra-peritoneal injection (into the abdominal cavity). Firstly, the affinity of the haematoxylin to the tumour tissue was so pronounced that it made its way from the abdominal cavity to the cancer cells lying below the skin. No other healthy organ or tissue structures were marked. Secondly, the electron microscope images of the large-cell lymphomas showed, surprisingly, that the intracellular plasma had been destroyed. This extracellular matrix, however, is of vital importance for the provision and interaction of the (cancer) cells. When this nourishing infrastructure is removed, supply to the malignant tissue is cut off and it is starved. Be- *Cancer cells* cause the DMSO–haematoxylin mixture evidently only cuts off the *starved* supply to the tumorous tissue, the survival of the patient is ensured.

It can be deduced from Rogers' work that the DMSO–haematoxylin mixture causes an oxidative reaction with the 'acidic', anaerobic tumour cells. This reaction deactivates the intracellular matrix and starves the cancer cells to death. In this process DMSO assumes the important role of transport vehicle, ensuring that the haematoxylin is carried into the tissue effectively.

Tucker, who was insulted and called a heretic and a quack by col- *Unrecognised* leagues, was judged by his patients to be a hero. Morton Walker compares *geniuses* Tucker's courage in defying the wrath of his sceptics with the deeds of Louis Pasteur and Ignaz Semmelweis in the mid-nineteenth century. Pasteur postulated that severe illnesses were caused by bacteria, only to be mocked by his contemporaries. We now know that he was absolutely correct and it is hard to imagine that the mainstream medical establishment of his day was too ignorant to understand this.

Semmelweis drastically reduced the high mortality rate of young mothers suffering from childbed fevers by instructing the midwives in his clinic to wash their hands. This was the birth of hygiene regulations. The current German Wikipedia entry[64] explains: 'Semmelweis' discoveries were not recognised during his lifetime and were rejected by positivistically-minded critics and colleagues in particular as "speculative rubbish". Only a few doctors supported him; hygiene was generally regarded as a waste of time and to be incompatible with the prevailing theories on the cause of diseases.'

As a result, the Semmelweis case came to be regarded as being so *The Semmel-* important in the history of medicine that the so-called 'Semmelweis Re- *weis Reflex* flex' was named after him. The term is used to describe the human tendency to automatically react to groundbreaking innovations and their discoverers with scorn. The same source explains: 'The term "Semmelweis Reflex", according to which innovations in science are met with punishment rather than the appropriate reward because established paradigms and behavioural habits stand opposed to them, was coined by Robert Anton Wilson and named after Semmelweis.'

Lifesaver One of the patients whose life was saved by Tucker and his DMSO–haematoxylin mixture was a three-year-old boy suffering from an aggressively metastasising endothelioma. He had tumours on the inner wall (endothelium) of the blood and lymph vessels. Doctors at another hospital who were treating the boy for an additional illness (diabetes) withdrew treatment, furious that he was also taking alternative medicines. Tucker helped the child free of charge, and the other patients at his clinic made a collection to pay for the medication that the mother had to buy herself when the other hospital refused to help her. In this case DMSO–haematoxylin solution was administered orally. The boy was given five drops in purified water before breakfast.

In DMSO and haematoxylin as a combination treatment, it appears that we have another potent anti-cancer medicine at our disposal. It certainly deserves our attention as a cheap, and side effect-free, alternative to conventional medicine's chemotherapy.

Method Tucker gave the following suggestions regarding the dose and administration of his mixture:

25 grams of haematoxylin is dissolved in 75 millilitres of DMSO. The mixture is stirred until no sediment settles at the bottom. This stock solution is then ready for use. Haematoxylin is used as a cell dye in microscopy and is available from laboratory suppliers. However, always buy it in a pure powder form and not as a solution preparation, which often contains additives.

Injection / infusion: when the substance is taken intravenously, start with a dose of 1ml per 34kg (75 pounds) of body weight. However, it is better to begin treatment using an infusion consisting of 0.5ml DMSO–haematoxylin mixture in a 250ml 5% glucose solution infusion bottle. The drop rate should be set at less than 50 drops per minute so as to avoid causing irritation to the veins and to avoid the formation of blood clots. If that is tolerated well, the dose can be increased by 10% daily. According to Tucker the individual tolerance limit has been reached when, after the administration of a new, higher dose, the patient suffers a 30-minute fever. This is another reason why this kind of cancer treatment should only be carried out by doctors and alternative health practitioners who have sufficient experience to ensure the patient's safety and wellbeing. Tucker states that this temporary fever can be alleviated with a 50mg Benadryl® tablet, which is an anti-allergen and sedative containing the active component diphenhydramine. It is also available under the names Hevert-Dorm®, Dolestan®, Dormutil®, Emesan®, Halb-mond®, Moradorm®, Nervo OPT®, Sediat®, Sedopretten® and Vivinox-Sleep®. However, always read the information on the label regarding side effects and contraindications.

Oral administration: you can also drink the above mixture of the stock solution and 5% glucose solution. Only if the patient is suffering from stomach cancer should this not be done, as the treatment would cause the tumour to disappear too quickly, leaving a hole in the stomach. Stomach cancer should always be treated by infusion. About 60ml (2 ounces) of the glucose solution and the usual quantity of the DMSO–haematoxylin solution (1ml per 34kg body weight) is suggested for the drink mixture. This drink is taken in the morning on an empty stomach. Do not eat or drink for at least 30 minutes after taking the drink. Ideally the glucose would be replaced by some other substance that makes the taste milder, not only for diabetics but for all patients who want to make conscious nutritional choices. Possible alternatives include xylitol or a pinch of stevia extract, which you add to the aqueous DMSO–haema-toxylin solution.

Inhalation: to treat lung cancer, Tucker suggests filling an inhalator with a mixture of 2ml saline solution and 4 drops of the DMSO–haematoxy-lin stock solution. Inhale for 10 minutes twice a day. Leave at least two hours between sessions.

External application: Tucker explains the method of local application using the example of skin cancer on the face. A small quantity of the stock solution is mixed with the same volume of distilled water so that the concentration of the two active substances is halved. This solution is dabbed onto the affected areas of skin, using cotton swabs, twice a day. The concentration can be increased gradually if no allergic reaction is experienced.

Tucker recommends carrying out the respective application every day, and to check the CEA value of the blood once a month if it is elevated at the beginning, i.e. before treatment starts. The CEA is the carcino-embryonic antigen, which can be used as a general tumour marker to monitor the progress of the disease. Treatment should be continued until this value is below the normal range (< 4.6ng/ml; for smokers < 10ng/ml). Tucker states that alcohol and nicotine should be completely avoided during treatment. The patient should drink plenty of liquids and consume a high intake of vitamins.

2.5.4 DMSO and other (cancer) medications

The possibilities for combining DMSO with other medicinal substances are practically boundless. In conventional medicine it is common to combine DMSO with cortisone, antibiotics, painkillers and local anaesthetics.

DMSO not only increases the effectiveness of antibiotics (medications which fight bacteria) but also that of virustatics (virus inhibitors), antifungals (fungal inhibitors), and substances that kill other microorganisms. Increased effectiveness means, inversely, that lower doses can be administered. This effect is often highly desirable when the goal is to minimise the side effects of the listed substances as much as possible.

In many cases this method can bring long-term cortisone treatment doses down below the Cushing threshold, i.e. the quantity of cortisone that can lead to serious side effects when taken for more than two weeks. Incidentally, there is a whole range of potent anti-inflammatory alternatives to cortisone; these alternatives come without the side effects of cortisone, and include lipoic acid, ascorbate, sodium bicarbonate / procaine, vitamin B12 and DMSO itself.

DMSO's carrier function is unequalled, making new treatment approaches possible as a result. For example, the highly inadequate but widespread treatment for children suffering inflammation of the middle ear is systemic administration of antibiotic or penicillin as a juice. This is unnecessary. In some European countries this kind of treatment is even frowned upon because it carries the risk that the bacteria will develop a resistance. Irrespective of the fact that even conventional doctors are now increasingly taking a wait-and-see stance when treating this kind of infection, and are only administering ibuprofen as an anti-inflammatory, it can certainly be wise to use antibiotic medicines in individual or chronic cases. The solution is to mix DMSO with the antimicrobial substance and apply this to the ear canal. DMSO can transport the antimicrobial substance through the eardrum and into the middle ear. MMS / CDS and hydrogen peroxide are also effective anti-microbial substances and can be readily combined with DMSO for such purposes.

In addition to the mixtures of DMSO and the substances described in detail above, there are, from an alternative medicine perspective, a number of other interesting options that will be mentioned here only briefly. These combination options largely pertain to the treatment of cancer. *Anti-cancer* Very recent research has shown in a very impressive way that other *substances* molecules that are, biochemically speaking, small and that we have long known about promise excellent results when used to treat malignant tumours. All these substances are widely available to purchase – that is precisely the reason why the pharmaceutical industry does not carry out expensive clinical trials on them. It makes more business sense to 'push' the more expensive chemotherapy medications. The alternative substances include DCA (dichloroacetic acid), right-turning lactic acid, and alpha lipoic acid (coenzyme for oxidation reactions).

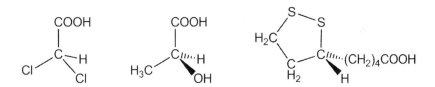

Figure 38: Molecule structure of DCA, S-(+)-lactic acid, and R-(+)-lipoic acid

An article addressing this issue in *Neue Zürcher Zeitung* (NZZ online, 2 April 2007) summarises the relevant results in a plain and easy-to-understand way. These three substances have long been used in the treatment of other illnesses. DCA has been used to treat the metabolic disorder lactic acidosis; S-(+)-lactic acid has been used to treat dysbiosis (disorder of the intestinal flora); alpha lipoic acid has been used to treat diabetic polyneuropathy (damage to the nerve cells), liver disease and heavy metal poisoning (chelation therapy). That means that we have much experience to draw from regarding the use of these three substances in humans.

Although there may not be an obvious common denominator in the above list of fields of applications, what we have covered so far may help you to understand why these substances are effective cancer treatments.

Mitochondria They influence the metabolism of the cells by normalising the mitochon-
regulators dria function, i.e. they restore normal cell respiration and promote the
process of programmed cell death, or make it possible where it had
ceased to occur. That is why these substances so quickly and convincingly
won their place in the field of alternative cancer therapy. In my opinion
we should regard official reports on the harmful effects of these three
substances, as well as the warnings against taking them on your own responsibility, as coming from a commercial and business context. Who
could derive any advantage if you treat yourself, and cheaply at that?

When the dosage recommendations and the guidelines for use are
observed, these are very safe medicines. After all, lactic acid and lipoic
acid have been in use and marketed pharmaceutically for many years.
How can these substances suddenly be dangerous simply because they
are administered to treat a different disease?

Let us now return to our main topic, which is the combination of such
medicines with DMSO. By themselves, these substances may not have
had the hoped-for medicinal effect, and you may be confronted with the
question of whether to increase the dose or whether there may be another
way to improve the effect. You can surely guess the answer! These are all
substances that must be transported into the cells of the affected tissue so
that they can unleash their pharmacological properties. Only then can
they influence the mitochondria and the metabolic processes. What substance can transport them there? DMSO, of course, the universal carrier.

Dichloroacetic Evangelos Michelakis' in-vitro and animal experiments present a strong
acid case for the use of **dichloroacetic acid** as an anti-cancer medication. He
suggests a starting dose of 10mg per kg of body weight per day (e.g. 0.7g/d
for a person weighing 70kg). DCA has a long biological half-life of one
day and therefore need not be administered every day. There is a host of
tips, instructions and formulas on the website www.thedcasite.com ('The
DCA Site'), all provided by people who have used DCA themselves. They
advise taking DCA for 5 days, then taking a break of 2 days. They recommend diluting DCA in water and drinking it.

However, we know that DCA is not particularly soluble and that it
can have quite an irritating effect in this form. It can remain in the stomach as a free acid and is therefore not resorbed. Is there a solution for
this? DCA must be carried into the tissue and the cells. It is readily soluble in DMSO. Any other questions?

Various media reports have warned against taking DCA because it can cause trembling, fatigue and pain when taken in large quantities or for long periods. Not everyone experiences these symptoms and they are fully reversible according to observations made so far. You can determine your individual tolerance limit by carefully observing yourself and your response as you take this substance.

Right-turning lactic acid has, essentially, been used therapeutically for *Right-turning* millennia. As a 'by-product' of fermentation processes, such as in the *lactic acid* preservation of sauerkraut for example, its positive effects on digestion and on the immune system have long been known. Lactic acid is formed through the metabolic activity of Lactobacteria such as the well-known strains *Lactobacillus casei* and *Lactobacillus bulgaricus*. These natural processes do not produce pure S-lactic acid (also called L-(+)-lactic acid) but a mixture of the S and the R form (also called D-(-)-lactic acid). The difference between the two lies in the arrangement of the ligands around the central C-atom. The structures represent an opposite reflection of one other. You may remember the pyramid-shaped structure of the sulfoxides discussed in the 'Chemical properties' section. Whenever a carbon atom in the centre of such a pyramid is surrounded by four different ligands (i.e. other atoms or groups of atoms), we are dealing with the phenomenon of chirality or enantiomerism.

The term chirality comes from the Greek and is often translated as *'Right and left'* 'handedness'. This means that the two molecular forms of the same compound differ in the same way that our left and right hands differ. As geometric figures they cannot be made congruent even though they are, in terms of their make-up, the same substance. As a point of comparison: because the DCA molecule carries two identical atoms around the central carbon atom, you do not find a mirror image there (see figure 38).

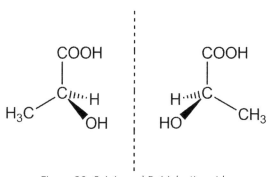

Figure 39: S-(+)- and R-(-)-lactic acid

131

The different molecule structures, having four different neighbours arranged around one carbon atom, really do lead to measurable differences in terms of the physical and biochemical properties of the mirror image substances. These substances have been named after their ability, in a solution, to rotate the plane of polarised light clockwise or anti-clockwise. That is what is meant by 'right-turning' and 'left-turning'. This change can be identified relatively easily with the aid of a suitable lamp and two polarisation films. Such experiments are perfect for biology or physics lessons.

The phenomenon of chirality is common in nature, i.e. organic substances (carbon compounds) are often found in a pure R- or S- form, known as chiral enantiomers. Examples of these include DNA, amino acids, proteins and carbohydrates (e.g. cellulose, starches, etc.). In this respect evolution has led to a far-ranging selectivity or preference for only one of the two mirror images in each respective case. On a macroscopic level we see this from the fact that snail shells are usually formed in a right-turning spiral, for example. It is often the case that substances of animal or plant origin are actually only effective or viable in one, naturally-occurring left- or right-turning form. All living creatures are, ultimately, enantiomeric structures because they are selectively built from chiral molecules. That is why reverse-image substance particles can evoke recognisability through the sensory cells. A lovely example of this is the etheric oil carvone. Its right-turning S-form smells like caraway and has an LD_{50} value of 3.6g/kg (rats). The left-turning R-form smells like mint and has an LD_{50} value of 1.6g/kg (rats), and is therefore significantly more toxic.

A marvel of nature

The world of medicine has also had to learn the bitter lesson that this is also true of artificially produced 'laboratory substances'. It became clear, at a very high human cost, that the left-turning thalidomide (Contergan®) led to abnormalities in unborn children whereas the right-turning form did not. Since the product was produced synthetically, both variants were formed unselectively as a 50:50 mixture. This is also called a racemate. The retrospective separation of such laboratory-produced substances into two pure enantiomers is usually very intensive work in terms of time, materials and cost. Because of that, intensive research work is being undertaken across the world in a bid to discover enantioselective syntheses, i.e. production processes for pure R- or S-compounds.

Even today, companies often shy away from the effort involved in separating 50:50 mixtures for the production of synthetic medications. That is the case, for example, with the 'stomach protection' medicine pantoprazole. It belongs to the group of stomach acid-inhibitors (PPIs / proton pump inhibitors such as omeprazole, lansoprazole) and is a 50:50 enantiomer mixture from both mirror-image forms. These days this medication is even advertised as an over-the-counter treatment for stomach ulcers and inflammation of the oesophagus. The enantiomers are not separated (except for Nexium®).

Why are these medications relevant? From a chemical perspective the PPIs belong, as does DMSO, to the sulfoxides group. However, that inconsequential fact is the only thing these two substance classes have in common because the PPIs consist of significantly larger molecules that have more complex structures. I strongly advise against thoughtlessly consuming these stomach acid inhibitors. Even if the label 'stomach protection' may sound harmless (who introduced that, I wonder?) the substance seriously interferes with digestive regulation and acid–alkaline balance in general. It would be quite foolish to assume that the only place in the human body where 'proton pumps' are to be found is in the stomach wall. The body has to maintain a balance in a number of organs and tissue by actively transporting positively charged hydrogen ions (H^+). Through this process, bicarbonate anions (HCO_3^-) travel in a countercurrent to the other side of the biological membrane and chloride anions (Cl^-) passively diffuse. This is an extremely important and highly complex synergy of concentration dependencies that should not be put in danger by taking PPIs thoughtlessly, or on a long-term basis.

Nature does it best! Biological syntheses and metabolic processes are reg- *Nature as* ulated by enzymes (our biocatalysts) that are also chiral; these processes *teacher* usually proceed highly selectively as a result. That is why the S-(+)-lactic acid is the only natural variant tolerated by the human body and it also occurs as a metabolic product. It is therefore also called an eutomer in this context.

In contrast, our bodies struggle to cope with the non-physiological R-(-)-lactic acid (distomer). It is more difficult to break down, excretion is slow and it can accumulate in the tissue. It has a coagulant effect and therefore impairs the viscosity of the blood and lymph. It binds to minerals such as calcium, iron and selenium so that it can be eliminated, meaning that valuable nutrients are lost as a result. It can also bind to uric acid and cholesterol, leading to the formation of molecular complexes that are not readily soluble and which, as deposits, cause rheumatic and arteriosclerotic problems. So if you are taking lactic acid as part of a nutritional supplementation programme, you should make sure that the product contains as much right-turning S-lactic acid as possible.

Unfortunately, lactobacteria do not produce lactic acid according to the process of selectivity described above. Depending on the strain of bacteria, the concentration of the S-form lies at between 50 and 90%, which must then be purified. The right-turning lactic acid products commonly sold at pharmacies and health food shops are usually approximately 20% liquid solutions. When taking such a concentrate you should bear in mind that it is a strong organic acid that can in some cases cause damage to teeth. It should therefore always be heavily diluted in another liquid (water, fruit juice, tea) before being consumed. You will find a wide range of different dosage recommendations in the literature. Starting doses of 1ml of a 20% solution x 3 times a day appear to be reasonable (one-third to one-half of this amount for children).

Expect a range of therapeutic effects. They include more efficient elimination of the left-turning lactic acid, increased adrenalin activity, improved acid–alkaline balance and better viscosity of the blood and lymph.

Effective cancer cell inhibitor As a result of their anaerobic energy production, cancer cells in particular produce large amounts of left-turning lactic acid. This weakens the surrounding tissue and promotes the spread of malignant tumours. Because the S-lactic acid, in contrast, promotes aerobic metabolic processes, the renegade cells can return to normal mitochondrial activity and programmed cell death processes become activated. It is still unclear whether this can be attributed to the direct influence of the resorbed S-lactic acid. Otto Warburg, the Nobel Prize winner mentioned earlier, theorised that the S-lactic acid absorbed from food predominantly unleashed its positive effect by improving the intestinal environment. Today, it is assumed that the 'good' intestinal bacteria such as *Lactobacillus* and *bifidus* produce butyrate – an effective cancer cell inhibitor. Moreover, healthy intestinal flora supports the detoxification and deacidification processes, thereby reducing the toxic load on our perpetually strained livers.

All these processes are dependent on the exchange of substances between the matrix and the cells functioning smoothly. The necessary diffusion processes can be supported (or made possible again) by administering DMSO in parallel. The combination of DMSO and S-(+)-lactic acid is recommended because it improves the absorption of the effective substance and the exchange of substances in the tissue, increasing the pressure on sick cells.

Lipoic acid is also a natural chiral substance and an integral part of the *An important* mitochondrial metabolism of all higher animals. The cellular power sta *coenzyme* tions depend on the presence of this substance, although only the R-(+)-enantiomer, the alpha lipoic acid, is biologically active. It functions as a coenzyme in oxidative reactions. In the process, as a result of the splitting of the sulphur–sulphur bond (disulphide), it is reduced to R-dihydrolipoic acid before finally being reformed following a recycling stage. When supplied from external sources the dihydrolipoic acid appears to have greater therapeutic effect.

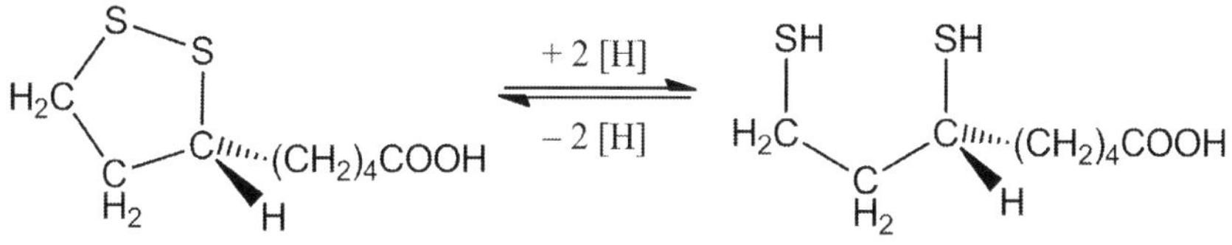

Figure 40: Redox balance between R-lipoic acid and R-dihydrolipoic acid

The body needs alpha lipoic acid to regenerate expended radical scavengers and antioxidants such as vitamin C, vitamin E, coenzyme Q10 and glutathione. It can also be used as a binder in chelation treatments for heavy metal toxicity. Alpha lipoic acid also stimulates the synthesis and release of the nerve growth factor – that is why it is used in cases of peripheral neuropathy in diabetes patients.

Of much greater importance in this context, however, is the fact that the substance can regenerate and influence the mitochondria activity of cancer cells. As explained above, this leads to the repression of anaerobic cell processes and to the stimulation of the intended death of sick cells. It looks unlikely that the pharmaceutical giants or the universities *Mitochondria* will carry out further clinical trials because lipoic acid, like the other *switch* substances discussed above, has long been available off-patent. We can, therefore, use it whenever we wish and use this substance to demonstrate that experiential alternative medicine, alongside institutionalised pharmaceutical research, makes an important contribution to the health of the populace.

Proof of the effect of lipoic acid on metabolic processes in mitochondria was provided in a 2005 publication by Professor Hannelore Daniel

(TU Munich, Chair in Nutritional Physiology) and Professor Uwe Wenzel, who teaches and researches at the Institute of Molecular Nutritional Research, Justus-Liebig Universität Giessen.[66] Their work demonstrates clearly how the energy production centres that have been shut down in cancer cells are 'switched on' again, in the sense that normal cell respiration and the resulting cellular life cycle is resumed.

You can buy alpha lipoic acid in tablet or capsule form at any pharmacy. The therapeutic effect is noticeable at doses from about 50mg per day. However, general dose recommendations are usually set at 250mg to 750mg. Tablets and injection ampules containing 600mg of R-lipoic acid are common, although the ampules are significantly more expensive. One gram of lipoic acid in tablet form can cost as little as 50 pence from internet retailers. The 600mg tablets should be taken in the morning, half an hour before breakfast. To combine it with DMSO, you can drink the DMSO dissolved in water when taking the lipoic acid or take it after breakfast as usual.

2.5.5 DMSO and ascorbic acid

Natural deficiency Ascorbic acid is better known by the name 'vitamin C'. This substance is hugely important for the health of the human body, as we have only recently begun to fully understand. The flood of scientific research and the (often wrongly interpreted) information published in the media is overwhelming. Unlike most other living beings primates, including humans, cannot produce this essential vitamin internally themselves. Ingestion from food via the intestinal mucosa is only possible to a limited extent and large quantities of it (> 200mg) fail to reach the bloodstream via this route. The physiological reabsorption rate in the renal tubules is also rather low.

On the whole, this is less than optimal for us when we consider that long-term deficiency leads to death. In contrast, bacteria, vertebrates and plants can produce ascorbic acid via their metabolic processes by converting the ubiquitous molecular building blocks glucose or galactose whenever they need. Some studies have even shown that the ascorbic acid production, or the quantity of vitamin C present in the blood (plasma concentration), of various animals rises as their stress levels rise. This is an indication that this substance determines and promotes the capacity of an organism to perform.

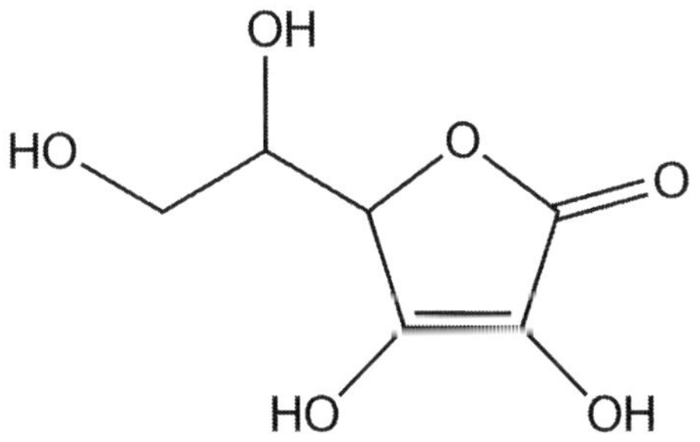

Figure 41: Ascorbic acid / vitamin C

The amazing treatment results we acquire today from high-dose ascorbic acid treatment can only be achieved with infusions, thereby bypassing the gastrointestinal tract. Ascorbic acid infusions are given to treat the symptoms of old age, pain in the musculoskeletal system, infections, stress, burnout, inflammations, allergies, and tumours, as well as following operations or for high-level sportspeople. Sadly, it is often only wealthy private patients or famous sportspeople who benefit from this treatment because the German medical system refuses to meet the cost. Fortunately, however, ascorbic acid infusions can be obtained at relatively low prices, meaning that anyone earning the average wage can afford this highly effective treatment. *Vitamin C, the all-rounder*

Based on the extensive experience gathered by specialised therapists, we know that the list of therapeutic fields of application is very long. This demonstrates that ascorbic acid, like DMSO, has a comprehensive and universal regulation effect on the body. Unlike DMSO, however, there is a specific illness that results from vitamin C deficiency – scurvy. Its symptoms include immune system weakness and infirm connective tissue. Other symptoms include reduced energy, joint pain, susceptibility to infection, slow wound healing and reduced elasticity of the blood vessels. In addition, a type of anaemia can manifest itself which, under laboratory analysis, appears similar to iron deficiency anaemia. The red blood cell count is extremely low and the cells that are present are too small and 'pale' (hypochromic, microcytic anaemia). The fragility of the blood cells can, in extreme cases, lead to damage to the vessel walls, resulting in internal bleeding.

Based on this information, you will surely be able to work out why vitamin C is used in the treatment of the above mentioned diseases and for regeneration and energy improvement. This comprehensive treatment concept has been and is predominantly being developed and taught by the Pascoe company based in Giessen, Germany. The Pascoe product Pascorbin® is the only high-dose vitamin C solution approved for infusion therapy that is widely available as a medical preparation. It contains 7.5 grams of ascorbic acid dissolved in 50 millilitres of liquid.

Medical practitioners can also order tailor-made solutions at special pharmacies. What is interesting here is that we can manage the pharmacological activity spectrum by determining the total quantity administered and the infusion drop speed. This knowledge is more necessary when treating severe illnesses than less serious cases.

Pro-oxidative effect   And now we come to discuss combinations of ascorbic acid and DMSO – both of which are classed as antioxidants. While DMSO, despite that categorisation, promotes vital immunological oxidation processes by means of its ability to cross barriers and its modulation properties, ascorbic acid, above a certain quantity threshold, can even have a pro-oxidative effect of its own. Armed with these two protagonists, we have a wide range of healing effects because they work pro-oxidatively, but they can also be used as regenerative substances. Metaphorically speaking, you must first win the battle against microorganisms, toxins, tumour cells, etc. After that, however, it is important to undertake a clean-up operation to return the body to a state that is as close as possible to its natural, original condition. 'Scars' of all shapes and sizes (viewed holistically) may remain; they represent something akin to a structural memory on the physical level.

Whenever I hear the word 'scars' I am always reminded of images of enormous whales, the visible surface of whose bodies are often covered by countless battle scars. These scars bear witness to heroic battles for survival in the depths of the sea and they seem to me to be a biography recorded, not digitally but multidimensionally, in the tissue.

But let us return to the applications of DMSO and ascorbic acid. While infusion is the only suitable way of administering a targeted delivery of vitamin C, DMSO can be given as a drink solution, applied externally to *Synergies* the skin, or as an infusion. Taken together the two substances are excellent for promoting healing, detoxification and regeneration processes in equal measure and are mutually supportive. As far as I am aware, no scientific studies have been carried out on the potential reciprocal effects on cell uptake, metabolism or elimination rate. Simultaneous use, as is the case with the previously mentioned combination examples, is still exclusively based on the experience of alternative medical practitioners and their patients. But since we have extensive scientific data on both substances individually, we can predict potential reciprocal effects. We know, for example, that the oxidised form of ascorbic acid, dehydroascorbic acid (DHA), normally uses the same transport systems as glucose for cell uptake. Elevated blood sugar values therefore lead to reduced uptake, which obviously exacerbates problems in cases of diabetes (or in general regarding obesity and overeating today). When taken with DMSO the penetration of cell membranes is made much easier. We humans have specific transport proteins in the cell membranes for the sodium salt of ascorbic acid, sodium ascorbate. DMSO, because it improves solubility, also aids the elimination of ascorbic acid, ascorbate and other metabolic products such as DHA and oxalic acid via the kidneys.

Another example of the complementary functions of DMSO and vitamin C can be found in the area of collagen synthesis and the regulation of this process. Chapter 1.2.3 'Pharmacological properties' has already outlined how DMSO modulates collagenase activity and can have a positive effect on potentially excessive repair work in the connective tissue. Ascorbic acid is essential for the structurally selective formation of collagen because it makes it possible for an amino acid (proline) to transform into its oxidised form. Only then do the giant collagen molecules obtain their spatially fixed, three dimensional form. The synergy between DMSO and ascorbic acid is therefore particularly useful when treating injuries, symptoms of old age, and following operations.

These suggestions and examples of possible combinations are intended to encourage you to exploit your understanding of the principles of DMSO use in order to gather your own new experiences. With time you will develop your own unique way of using this treatment and you will never want to be without it. As long as you bear in mind the safety instructions, which have been repeated many times here, you can experiment to your heart's content – as many other patients and therapists have discovered. There are some who use DMSO in combination with homeopathic or plant medicines. There are others who use the procaine–DMSO mixture (or lidocaine and others) as a needle-free alternative to neural or acupuncture treatment. Others combine DMSO with natural amino acid sources such as algae or cereal grasses to prepare medications that can be hugely beneficial to hyperactive or developmentally delayed children. DMSO is also sometimes combined with a standard diclofenac preparation (e.g. Diclac®, Voltaren® as a gel) and used externally as a fortified application of this antirheumatic agent (see heel spur, Chapter 3). You can be creative – both for yourself and for your patients!

FIELDS OF APPLICATION AND CASE EXAMPLES

This chapter lists and describes the many diseases and complaints that have been successfully treated using DMSO. One of DMSO's astounding properties as a superordinate therapeutic principle is that many of these diseases have, at first glance, no common denominator. This list is naturally not comprehensive and new fields of application for DMSO and its special pharmacological properties will always be discovered. If you have experience of working with DMSO we would be delighted to hear from you and I will include such information in any future editions of this book. Bear in mind that you cannot assume that positive treatment results experienced by some patients can be automatically reproduced in all patients. Take your responsibilities towards yourself and others seriously and seek help from experienced doctors or alternative health practitioners, who can diagnose severe illnesses by taking the case history, undertaking physical examinations and giving advice. In addition, do not forget to carry out the mandatory tolerance test before you use DMSO on yourself or others for the first time.

When different application methods are mentioned in this chapter (e.g. oral or external application), you can turn back to Chapter 2, where you will find instructions and starting dose recommendations. These too are recommendations based on experience and we cannot assume that they will be valid for everybody. With some practice you can develop your own 'style' and follow your own path.

Accidents / whiplash

Even when there are no visible signs of injury, rear-end collisions can cause serious health problems. The term 'whiplash' covers injuries to the head, neck, shoulders and torso. The force generated in (car) accidents produce movements in the musculoskeletal structure that go beyond the normal range of movement. Bruising and contusions can result. Long-term joint damage is only one of the possible consequences, especially in the cervical spine. The main symptom is severe pain over a number of days, often exacerbated by movement. Other possible complaints include neuropathological symptoms such as headaches, dizziness, unsteady gait, and speech difficulties. The body is urgently working on the repair and regeneration of strained and injured physical structures. Patients sometimes feel feverish and exhausted.

The scientific literature indicates a range of different statistics regarding those who go on to develop chronic complaints. Some state that the figure is 60%, while others say that the high number of cases that are (allegedly) never cured can be partly accredited to people hoping for compensation and time off work. It appears that wearing a neck brace (and the limited movement / relieving posture associated with them) leads to long-term problems more often than is the case when the patient undergoes movement therapy at the earliest opportunity. The muscle relaxants that are often prescribed as a parallel treatment can be highly addictive (the first step towards tranquilizer addiction). Another factor that can contribute to whiplash injuries becoming chronic (i.e. symptoms persisting for a period longer than 6 months) is failure to adequately process the psychological trauma of the accident and the resulting injury. Listening attentively as the patient discusses such issues is far more helpful than prescribing popular painkillers.

DMSO makes it possible for us to successfully and holistically treat whiplash and bruising resulting from accidents. Pain relief, muscle relaxation, regeneration, tissue detoxification, cell stabilisation – this substance provides all these effects and is well tolerated. When DMSO is used early, the patient avoids the need to adopt relieving or improper postures and the body's natural movement patterns can return. You can do without the neck brace. Ideally, DMSO should be applied locally to the skin and, at the same time, taken internally as a drink solution or infusion.

Case:[19] Marvin Combs, then 66 years old and still very active as a building contractor, had a car accident in which he suffered whiplash. He had severe pains in his neck and in both arms, and his legs became very tender. Previous health conditions such as his arthritis were aggravated. The painkillers that were initially prescribed did not achieve the desired effect. But Marvin Combs did experience significant reduction in both the severe neck pains and his other problems after taking DMSO. Because the accident claim was to be heard in court he had to return to his original doctors. This meant that he had to stop taking DMSO since it was not officially approved as a medication. The patient was frustrated by the high costs of (private) treatment and by the ineffectiveness of the numerous tablets he had been prescribed. Once the accident claim was settled he immediately restarted the DMSO treatment. His medical record states that he was completely free of pain and sleeping like a baby after only five days of intravenous DMSO treatment. Before that he had still been suffering serious problems as a result of the accident. After that single week of treatment he was able to return to his normal work routine.

Achilles tendinitis

This chronic condition, which is usually extremely painful, is caused by overuse of, and placing improper strain on, the joint. In some cases, however, the tendon becomes inflamed spontaneously.

Treatment using DMSO: apply a 75% DMSO solution generously to the affected area. In acute cases this can be done two or three times a day. Always ensure that the solution has been completely absorbed before you wear socks / shoes.

Morton Walker[19] describes the case of the world-class 800m runner Morgan Growth, whose tendon condition was quickly healed using DMSO even though he had been plagued by it for a long while.

Acne

These inflammatory pustules, which are not only a problem for pubescent teenagers, can be soothed very effectively by dabbing them with DMSO solution. Facial skin usually reacts more sensitively to DMSO than other areas so begin treatment by using a 50% solution. The concentration can be increased to 75% if the initial tingling or itching is tolerated well. Just a few applications are usually sufficient to put a halt to emerging spots. We have had some very good results using it on our children.

It is possible to augment this DMSO treatment by applying hydrogen peroxide solution locally, or by administering lactic acid bacteria or effective microorganism preparations internally. I also like to use suspensions of suitable bacteria strains, together with fermented parts, directly on the skin. This leads to astounding reductions in acne and other skin inflammations. It is a shame that hardly anyone makes home-made sauerkraut these days. The liquid produced during the process would, at room temperature, be an ideal substance that has this fermentation effect, and it contains plenty of 'good' bacteria and lactic acid. As a child growing up in the provinces I belonged to the generation that was 'allowed' to help in the annual tradition of preparing sauerkraut in large earthenware pots. Back then there was limited enthusiasm for the work and now the knowledge has been lost.

Addiction See Withdrawal symptoms

ADHD See Developmental disorders in children

Ageing

(Premature) ageing leads to a number of conditions. These include problems with the skin (liver spots, wrinkles), organ dysfunction (reduced digestive or elimination capacity, impotence, etc.), limited nerve function (causing memory problems or neuropathies), and hair loss. In my opinion any anti-ageing programme deserving of its name should – alongside the main building blocks of nutrition, exercise / movement and sleep – include individual treatment methods that correspond to the patient's particular constitution. These may include detoxification / cleansing, parasite removal, deacidification, intestinal cleansing, interference field therapy and, if necessary, weight reduction. As an agent that has a comprehensive regenerative effect, DMSO has an important role to play as part of these anti-ageing measures. Taken internally, it breaks down hardened tissue, improves the effectiveness of the other programme elements and, as a diuretic, promotes the elimination of toxins via the kidneys. If you decide to make fundamental lifestyle changes in an attempt to regain your vitality, use DMSO in the early stages of rejuvenation work to stimulate important physical processes.

The extensive range of products offered on the anti-ageing and weight loss markets often leads to confusion and wasted money. In many cases pure lies are disseminated in an attempt to make a profit. You are probably familiar with the age-old fairy tale of the wonderful properties of 'diet' or 'sugar-free' drinks (Zero, Light), and of 'healthy spinach', or the lies regarding the 'dangers of lactose intolerance'. When you consider the natural physiology of the human body, most of these statements are completely worthless and misguided.

The problems of old age and excess weight are best tackled using simple, natural medicinal methods that are cheap and which make logical sense. Seek holistic advice and judge any recommended measure on its simplicity and on how close it is to what evolution had in mind for us hominids – certainly not facelifts and Botox injections. If you find yourself receiving advice from a medical practitioner who wants to 'sell' you an anti-ageing programme, you should perhaps consider whether her / his appearance reveals whether she / he has mastered the art of using natural measures for rejuvenation purposes. Personally I would not pay anyone who appears to be overweight or who has aged prematurely to advise me on rejuvenation and weight loss. A thorough understanding of physical processes (biological rhythms, hormone effects e.g. insulin, cell and organ function) almost automatically leads us to take a sensible course of action that supports rather than exploits and prematurely ages the body.

Learn from evolution   When long-term overeating leads to an illness such as diabetes, it is essentially the result of overstraining, exploiting and prematurely ageing the pancreas and the body's cells. The pancreas' response, quite naturally, is loss of function. That is the exact definition of ageing: a gradual decline in the function of the organs and tissue. Once we understand how the metabolic processes involved in this work, it becomes instantly clear that evolution has prepared us for days of want, not for days of plenty. Eating and digestion should be understood first and foremost as an acute strain on the body, a strain that should be mitigated in every way possible. As long as we associate prosperity with excessive supplies of industrially modified foodstuffs we will continue to cause our bodies lasting harm. That is why any serious anti-ageing programme should always include an element of fasting and / or nutritional change. In other words, anyone who eats a natural diet will only rarely need to look for a rejuvenation, vitality or weight loss programme. Because an understanding of these simple contexts and interrelationships forms the basis for a good life, I personally consider attending an in-person course (rather than a large event / class) to become an alternative health practitioner to be the best possible investment in your health – even if you have no intention of earning a living in this way. The benefits for you and for your personal development are substantial because you will acquire unbiased medical knowledge uninfluenced by the marketing machines of the nutritional supplement companies and the pharmaceutical and cosmetic industries; all this outside the limiting confines and stifling structures of mainstream medicine.

Age-related macular degeneration (AMD)

This eye disease causes gradual damage to the retina, emanating from the pigment epithelium and the choroid in the centre of the visual field, also known as the macula (yellow spot). As a rule, it is 'only' the centre of the visual field that is affected by the deterioration in eyesight, but this means that reading ability is particularly affected. This causes significant suffering for the patient, even if they are still able to find their way around even in poor light. Other symptoms include poor colour perception, reduced ability to adjust to bright and dark surroundings, and a tendency to be dazzled by bright lights. The main 'accepted' risk factors for this condition are age (usually over 50 years old), smoking and high blood pressure. Based on many years of research, however, Professor Emeritus Siegfried Hünig (University of Würzburg) has come to the conclusion that increased exposure to UV light and the higher 'blue light' levels in modern office lighting are also significant factors that cause AMD.[67] This is particularly true for people with blue or grey eyes because of a pigment deficiency that results in reduced UV protection. The natural, brown melanin pigments normally function as highly effective UV light filters. The problem concerns the shortwave aspects of sunlight below 385nm that are not captured by the statutory regulations governing sunglasses in most European countries. Professor Hünig and his son have therefore developed their own low-cost sunglasses that comply with the more stringent Swiss standards. Poor modern-day dietary habits are also a significant risk factor. Since we are dealing here with an age-related condition, the number of diagnosed cases is rising sharply as the average age of the population rises.

The aetiological cause is presumed to be oxidative damage in the area of the tissue membrane that is responsible for the movement of liquids and substances to and from the sensory cell layer of the eye. The tissue responds to the resulting metabolic limitations, as always, by regenerating the vessels. The flooding of these additional capillary branches ultimately leads to loss of sight in the macula area. Laser-based photocoagulation procedures can be used to burn these abnormal blood vessels – a treatment that limits the development of the condition. Pharmaceutical medications are also being researched and developed across the globe. These medications work by inhibiting or blocking the natural biochemical vascular endothelial growth factors. However, it appears that the medications developed so far can only slow down the development of the disease.

Because AMD is caused by oxidative processes, DMSO, which works as an antioxidant and as a regenerative agent, immediately suggests itself as an obvious treatment. This is supported by a number of studies that demonstrate how other antioxidants such as omega-3 fatty acids, zinc, carotene and vitamins C and E also have a positive effect on the condition. Another indication is the observation I have made that patients who take DMSO sometimes report an improvement in their eyesight as an unexpected but pleasant side effect. In one case this led to a female patient reporting with great surprise that she no longer needed her glasses the next morning. DMSO must be taken internally when treating age-related macular degeneration. This can be done by following the procedures already described: moistening large areas of the skin with a 70% solution, oral intake as a diluted drink solution, or infusion.

Allergies

Depending on the immune processes involved, allergies are divided into four categories (Type 1 to Type 4), each with its respective subcategories. We speak of an 'immediate' type, an 'immune complex' type, and a 'delayed' type. A range of illnesses are included such as atopic complaints, thyroid diseases / Graves' disease, rheumatic fever, ITP (explained below), baker's or farmer's lung, and nickel allergy. Ultimately, these diseases are all caused by an inappropriate (over-)reaction by individual elements of our multifaceted immune system, which is usually able to distinguish very precisely between 'innate' and 'alien' and has perfectly matched or dosed defence strategies at the ready. Those elements of the immune system that ensure that the defence measures underway can also be withdrawn or controlled are equally important. It is exactly these processes that usually become dysfunctional in allergic reactions.

Without having to further expand on the scientific aspects, we will recall that DMSO also has a modulating effect (i.e. balancing and regulating) on immunological processes. We see this clearly when allergic reactions such as atopic dermatitis (see Atopic dermatitis) react well to DMSO treatment. This positive effect on excessive immune reactions can be observed both in very acute cases (see Insect bites) and in chronic cases such as collagenosis ('soft-tissue rheumatism', see Rheumatism). A number of illnesses are listed in Chapter 3 that are understood to be caused by allergic processes. The recommended DMSO application method for each respective illness can be found in the relevant section.

Alzheimer's disease See Neurodegenerative disorders

Amyotrophic lateral sclerosis See Neurodegenerative diseases

Angina pectoris See Arteriosclerosis

Aphthae

Aphthae are ulcers (usually less than 1cm in size) on the mucous membrane of the oral cavity or the genital area. They become red and inflamed around the edges and have a white fibrinous membrane. Many patients complain of severe pain and swelling in the related lymph nodes, and an associated feeling of sickness. A number of factors are thought to cause the condition, among them a virus (herpes simplex), vitamin deficiency, stress, injuries, hormonal fluctuations, and chronic processes such as coeliac disease and inflammatory intestinal diseases.

Treatment using DMSO: take a 65 to 80% DMSO solution and dab it several times a day onto the affected areas using a cotton wool pad. If at all possible, allow the solution a few minutes to be absorbed before being wiped away by the tongue or saliva. Combinations with MMS or hydrogen peroxide can also be used in very persistent cases. Prepare a mouthwash in the usual concentration (e.g. 15 drops MMS or 1.5% hydrogen peroxide solution) and administer the mouthwash shortly before treating with DMSO. You could also mix both substances in an egg cup and dab it onto the skin immediately. If you decide to use that method, prepare the mixture freshly before each application. We have gathered together a number of positive experience reports from patients, demonstrating that aphthae and other inflammation sites in the mouth heal much more quickly using DMSO and the pain is significantly less.

Arteriosclerosis

Today, this condition is understood to include vascular hardening and deposits of various kinds, including fats, blood cells, calcium salts and connective tissue. These processes narrow the free lumen of the blood vessels, potentially leading to high blood pressure and insufficient blood supply to the organs and tissue. The most common consequences include heart attacks (narrowing of the coronary arteries), strokes (narrowing of the arteries in the brain) and peripheral artery occlusive disease or PAOD (narrowing of the arteries in the legs). Heart valve disease can also develop if deposits accumulate there. Meaningful attempts to treat arteriosclerosis, which naturally must include nutrition, exercise / move-ment and change in lifestyle, are usually only made after these 'life-threatening' illnesses have reared their ugly heads. DMSO has a vaso-dilatory effect, dissolves fats and other substances, loosens connective tissue and breaks down deposits. As a result, it is just as suitable for use to prevent arteriosclerosis from developing as it is to treat the results once it has taken hold. Patients who develop cerebral complications in connection with arteriosclerosis, strokes, senility, head injuries or neu-rodegenerative brain diseases also benefit greatly from DMSO treat-ment. You will find additional relevant information under 'Developmen-tal disorders in children'.

The best way to treat arteriosclerosis using DMSO is by infusion. Dose options were given in Chapter 2. Alternatively, DMSO can also be ad-ministered onto the skin or taken as a drink solution. Narrowed vessels lead to a permanent lack of oxygen in the body, felt particularly in the oxygen-hungry organs such as the heart, brain, and kidneys. It is there-fore advisable to simultaneously administer oxidative substances that im-prove oxygen supply to the tissue and improve the loading efficiency of the red blood cells. Such combinations of DMSO and oxidative sub-stances (CDS, H_2O_2) can be used to treat all circulation problems that arise in connection with arteriosclerosis. These include angina pectoris, elevated blood pressure, smoker's leg and brain dysfunctions. Depending on the concentrations used, DMSO and CDS / H_2O_2 should not be ad-ministered together in one infusion. It is easier to administer them at staggered intervals. Other substances that could be useful include right-turning lactic acid, magnesium chloride and MSM. Patients suffering from arteriosclerosis, particularly those who develop serious secondary diseases due to narrowing of the vessels, must understand that their 'home-work' is just as important as the treatment given using the medications listed above. A resolute shift to a natural diet and comprehensive lifestyle changes will be required. Alcohol, tobacco and processed sugar must be completely avoided, as should (pork) meat and milk. If you or your patient is prepared to do that, the treatment recommended above could really help to improve circulation throughout the whole body.

Arthritis / arthrosis

This is one of the main fields in which DMSO has been used. A number of different pathological joint processes are usually conflated under the term *arthritis*. In German, the term actually only covers inflammatory processes (indicated by the ending '-itis'). These primarily include joint inflammations caused by microbes (usually bacteria such as *Staphylococcus* or *Streptococcus*) and the rheumatoid forms (autoimmune processes). The international definition of the term includes non-inflammatory joint processes (e.g. caused by degeneration, arthrosis). If you cast your mind back to the pharmacological properties of DMSO (see Chapter 1.2.3), it will instantly become clear that it is a suitable treatment for all the listed joint problems. It has anti-inflammatory and antimicrobial effects, it has a modulating effect on the immune system and, as part of its regenerative properties, it prevents degenerative processes. Furthermore, DMSO assumes a function as a carrier of other substances, thereby improving the potentially deficient supply of nutrition to the cartilage tissue. It is irrelevant which joints are affected but in my practice we have mainly been treating knees, shoulders, ankles, fingers and spines.

Treatment using DMSO: external administration is a very effective method when individual joints become diseased. The affected joint is moistened, covering as large an area as possible with a 60 to 80% aqueous DMSO solution using a brush or spray. Bear in mind that the skin above the waistline usually responds more sensitively than the skin below the waistline. That means that you should start with lower concentrations (e.g. 60%) when treating the shoulder, for example, but one would normally use a 75% solution when starting treatment on an ankle joint. You can often achieve swift reduction in symptoms with just one application a day. Where necessary the effect can be intensified by administering 2 or 3 external applications a day or by giving multiple daily doses. In severe cases affecting multiple joints, higher blood levels of DMSO can be achieved by taking internal applications (drinks or infusions). Such treatments usually start with doses of 0.05 to 0.1g DMSO per kg of body weight and the dose can be increased gradually, depending on progress, up to 0.5 to 1g per kg of body weight.

Case example:[19] Ruth Lewis, then 64 years old, had been suffering from rheumatoid arthritis for over twenty years and could only walk with the aid of a Zimmer frame. She could not close her right hand completely because of the pain. She had consulted a number of specialists and diagnostic clinics and had undergone a number of different treatments, but with no success. To make matters worse she then injured her back and her doctor instructed her to remain in bed for at least six months. Ruth Lewis feared that she would never walk again if she did so, so her son and her husband took her to a clinic to undergo DMSO treatment. After only two and a half weeks of daily DMSO infusions she left the clinic without the support of any walking aids. She said: 'I cannot put into words what this drug has done for me. I highly recommend it. I saw many people come and go during my stay; all walked out well.'

Asthma

Asthma can occur both as an allergic (atopic form) and as a non-allergic, chronic inflammatory reaction of the bronchial mucosa. However, a mixture of both forms is the most common. Mainstream medicine maintains that asthma is incurable. As a result patients, mostly children, face years of treatment using questionable but prevalent 'inhalers'. The main varieties are cortisone and beta2-adrenergic agonists, both of which have long-term side effects. You should not allow this to happen to your children. The main priority in any treatment is the avoidance of trigger substances / factors. These can include medications (e.g. painkillers such as aspirin), cold air (always breathe through the nose when taking part in outside sports in winter), organic solvents (nail varnish, paint, glue, sealants, air fresheners, cleaning detergents, etc.), fine dust / smog, animal hair, and all other animal and plant allergens. Any underlying illnesses (e.g. infections or heartburn) that trigger the asthma should also be treated. There is a significant psychological aspect to asthma and the other atopic diseases eczema and hay fever. Problems in school or family crises could be triggers for children. In my opinion asthma should be treated using DMSO (anti-allergenic, anti-inflammatory), complemented with immune system modulation measures (intestinal cleansing, basic salts, lactic acid, etc.), nutritional measures, and breathing therapy.

Treatment using DMSO: asthma is treated systemically, meaning that DMSO is given orally, by infusion, or is applied by brush onto large areas of the skin. After undertaking the compulsory tolerance test, start treatment by giving 3.5ml DMSO (half as much for children) in a glass with a drink (water, lukewarm tea, heavily diluted juice) once a day. The quantity can then be increased until you reach approximately 10ml. Even higher quantities should either be spread over the course of the day or be given by infusion. You should also take 'rest days' or limit treatment to 14 days to begin with because the substance accumulates in the body. You can adjust your approach according to the progress you make and the reduction you see in your symptoms.

Case: L., 8 years old, suffered from lung complaints and his story was a typical one. Recurring infections year-round and allergic episodes meant that his treatment included the use of inhalers. He found these difficult to use and they were ineffective because he could not master the breathing technique necessary to use them. The doctors responded by prescribing ever-higher doses. The boy, a lively lad, displayed typical side effects such as trembling and agitation. His lung function remained severely limited and sensitive to allergens as before. On my advice the mother has been giving him a daily dose of DMSO at the recommended quantities for a week. At first, the intention was to reduce the dose of asthma medication. However, the lung mucosa has now stabilised – clearly an indication of DMSO's anti-allergenic potential. The runny nose and breathing are improving noticeably.

Athlete's foot

This condition predominantly involves a fungal infection that appears in the form of a group of small blisters on the sole of the foot. As the condition develops, the skin wrinkles, peels and becomes hardened. The condition often occurs in those who regularly wear tight-fitting sports shoes. Traditional treatment using antifungal agents is often not effective enough to cure the condition. MMS footbaths and / or a combination treatment of MMS and DMSO are more effective. DMSO use results in the antifungal agent (in this case MMS) being carried more quickly and deeply into the skin. Moreover, DMSO has its own therapeutic effects. This treatment can be carried out in a number of ways. You can brush the feet with DMSO and wait a few minutes until the skin has dried a little. Then place the feet in an MMS bath prepared beforehand (e.g. 20 drops of activated MMS). You could also spray the feet liberally with MMS solution and then brush DMSO onto them immediately afterwards. Choose whichever method you find best.

Atopic dermatitis (see also Asthma, Allergies)

Atopic dermatitis can quickly be soothed using a 40 to 65% DMSO solution. This can probably be attributed mainly to the anti-allergenic and anti-inflammatory effects of DMSO. To complement the use of DMSO as a first aid measure, all atopic diseases should be approached holistically if there is to be hope of a long-term cure. Nutrition, intestinal flora therapy, mental hygiene and herbs are therefore all important treatment options. Because a number of very effective treatments are available for atopic and allergic reactions more generally, it is advisable to prepare a set of individual guidelines for each patient. That gives patients suffering from dermatitis a sense of assurance as they use methods with which they may not be familiar, having previously only used cortisone or zinc creams.

It is best to administer DMSO solutions onto the inflamed skin locally using a spray to avoid having to touch the affected skin. It is also advisable to take DMSO internally as a drink or as an infusion. You will find starting dose suggestions in the relevant sections of Chapter 2. I have also had success in treating infants and children affected by atopic dermatitis without using DMSO. The initial, temporary skin irritations commonly observed in adults might cause children to scratch themselves even more. I therefore recommend local treatment using solutions that bring about immediate relief. These include herbal extracts from heartsease (*Viola tricolor*) and the common daisy (*Bellis perennis*), and / or fermentation preparations of special bacteria. You can use probiotic cultures (e.g. lactic acid bacteria) or the liquid preparations known as effective microorganisms (EM). MMS sprays are also a suitable treatment. However, my approach could be judged as being overcautious. In practice, there is nothing to stop you from using diluted DMSO solutions even on very young infants as long as you have carried out the obligatory tolerance test beforehand.

Attention deficit disorders See Developmental disorders in children

Back / intervertebral disc problems

The intervertebral discs consist of an outer fibrous ring and an inner gel-like centre, the nucleus pulposus. The latter has the function of a water cushion that absorbs jolts. After the body length ceases to grow at the age of about 20, the intervertebral discs are no longer directly supplied by the blood vessels, only indirectly via passive diffusion processes. The transition between wakefulness and sleep is, therefore, vitally important for the supply and elimination of substances to and from this part of the spinal column. During the day, as you stand and sit, gravity induces a pressure on the nucleus pulposus, which then releases water and substances which are dissolved in it. This causes us to shrink by between 1 and 3cm over the course of a day. At night, as we lie down, the disc can fill once again – this is its process of regeneration. In adults, nutrients and waste products must be transported via this exchange of fluid and this is a very sensitive process. It is well known that damage to the intervertebral discs is caused by overstraining and improper movement, but problems can also arise 'spontaneously' following a dose of flu, or during pregnancy. The damage leads, via swelling or tearing, to the nucleus pulposus protruding or slipping out. This, in turn, causes irritation to the spinal cord structures, which can manifest itself in a range of symptoms such as pain, deafness and incontinence. I am told by osteopaths, physiotherapists and holistic doctors that it has now become a prevalent opinion that herniated intervertebral discs, apart from a few exceptions, can generally heal spontaneously. An operation – of whatever kind – is often totally unnecessary. For spontaneous healing to occur it is important that passive, manual and gymnastic measures are taken to take the pressure off the intervertebral discs so that the spine is given an opportunity to regenerate itself. Regeneration can only take place through a process of diffusion with the liquids in the surrounding area. Dissolved nutrients / electrolytes are transported in and superfluous substances are transported out. What substance do we know of that is excellent at promoting the transportation of other substances through biological membranes? Of course: DMSO is able to penetrate through the fibrous ring (annulus fibrosus) to reach the structure of the nucleus pulposus, which contains high levels of fluid, thereby modulating the cluster structure and transporting dissolved particles.

If you have undergone an operation on your spine, whether unwisely or not, you can still use DMSO as a regenerative substance. Apply a 70% DMSO solution externally onto large areas of the affected part of the back every day. Take a drink solution or infusions if you wish to take even higher quantities of DMSO. In veterinary medicine, DMSO infusions are a common treatment for horses that suffer back problems. The case of one of my current patients can illustrate the course of a treatment.

Case: Mr M. F., 31 years old, suffered a problem with one of the intervertebral discs in the lumbar area directly after a major life event (a happy one as it happens). He attributed this to the fact that his work involved sitting behind a desk for long hours and the resulting lack of movement. The problem quickly deteriorated and he exhibited all the signs of having a trapped nerve, accompanied with an associated fear of moving in case this would exacerbate the problem. His doctor advised him to undergo an operation immediately. The operation was carried out within the week and went as planned. The subsequent rehabilitation phase proved to be fitful and long-drawn-out. Faced with this set of circumstances I advised the patient to treat the injury externally with DMSO and to take the substance internally at the same time. After taking 5 to 10ml DMSO internally and applying the substance externally to the affected area every day for about 2 weeks there were extremely positive developments. The young man described the regenerative processes by saying: 'I'm surprised to discover that I've been able to return to my natural patterns of movement and I'm no longer afraid of walking. The scar has also become much softer.'

Baker's cysts

Cysts more generally are fluid-filled sacs that can form in tissue for a number of different reasons. They are often caused by inflammations, infections or parasites. Baker's cysts, also called popliteal cysts, involve a swelling of the knee capsule in the hollow of the knee. This is usually caused by a previous injury to the joint (e.g. a sports injury), or by degenerative or inflammatory processes such as arthrosis or rheumatism. The excess joint fluid produced as a result is forced to find somewhere to go, so it forms a separate, flexible water blister. Surgical removal often does not cure the problem because that approach does not heal the pathological processes in the joint, and the swelling returns.

Treating the whole knee joint by applying DMSO solution externally has a dual effect. Firstly, it cures the joint diseases, listed above, that cause increased influx of joint fluids. Secondly, the treatment promotes diffusion and osmosis processes in the cyst, thereby causing the swelling to shrink.

Apply a 75% aqueous DMSO preparation liberally onto the whole knee joint with a brush, as described in Chapter 2. This treatment should be carried out once a day until the condition is permanently resolved.

Bladder infections See Urinary tract infections

Blisters and calluses

Exerting too much friction or force on the skin can cause injuries and calluses, particularly on the hands and feet. In terms of DMSO treatment, these conditions can be treated as scars. Accordingly, a DMSO solution in concentrations of between 60 and 75% is applied externally. The healing or softening of the skin that DMSO brings about is only permanent if the cause of the friction (e.g. wearing shoes that are too small) is also dealt with. I have often successfully used DMSO to treat blisters and calluses caused by repetitive movements in sport or gardening. It always effects a very quick cure. Because DMSO treatment stops patients from bursting the fresh, liquid filled blisters, there is also less risk of developing an infection or inflammation.

Borreliosis / Lyme disease

Today there are a number of different alternative treatments for this chronic bacterial infection. The truth of the matter is that borrelia bacteria are very persistent in a number of ways and systemic antibiotic treatment is either very protracted or largely unsuccessful. That is why I consider a combination of an oxidative bactericide (MMS, MMS 2 or hydrogen peroxide) and DMSO as a carrier to be the best option. This ensures that even the body tissue that only receives minimal nutrition or does so only through diffusion (bradytrophic tissue) – i.e. the favourite hiding places for borrelia bacteria in their various forms, stages and variants – is flooded with the oxidative substance. Moreover, borrelia bacteria belong to the gram-negative class of bacteria and they release endotoxins when they are destroyed. These endotoxins can cause inflammatory or allergic reactions and must be eliminated by the body. DMSO is known to support this detoxification process.

Treatment using DMSO and MMS: it is easiest to take the two substances separately. First drink the required quantity of MMS (start with 2 drops and then increase the dose) and shortly afterwards take the DMSO solution. If that is too much for you, prepare the MMS drink in accordance with the guidelines and then add the desired quantity of DMSO and drink this mixture immediately. While Jim Humble says MMS should be taken at least three times a day, one or two doses of DMSO per day are sufficient.

Case: Ms H. G., 65 years old, had been suffering for many years from a range of symptoms which were only diagnosed as chronic borreliosis at a very late stage. She suffered from sleep disorder, anxiety, wandering pains, reduced energy, severe joint problems and she was putting on weight. Blood tests then showed elevated borrelia titer. After her doctors failed to offer her a convincing treatment plan she decided to try treatment using 'Fuller's teasel' extracts. She soon noticed changes but was not cured. She then took MMS for a number of weeks, which triggered severe detoxification reactions and caused great strain. It was now, if it had not been so before, that healing this disease would be a challenge. Blood tests taken after MMS treatment indicated that the borreliosis had disappeared, although that is not necessarily conclusive evidence. We discussed her situation once again and I advised her to stop trying to fight the infection for a while and to concentrate instead on her joint problems, which continued to torment her. On my advice she applied DMSO locally onto her feet and knees, which were causing pain, every day. This quickly alleviated the pains and swelling and there was a marked improvement in her mobility. She then switched to taking DMSO internally as a drink solution because she had started to suffer from severe sciatica (possibly due to the gardening she did as a result of the recent improvements in mobility and activity). That first night, after taking only 2 x 4ml of DMSO in a glass of water, she had the most refreshing sleep she had had in years. We must now wait to see how her condition develops.

Bowel diseases (chronic inflammatory)

The two most common chronic bowel diseases that involve detectable inflammation in the intestinal wall are ulcerative colitis and Crohn's disease. These diseases are distinguished by different histological characteristics diagnosed during a bowel examination, and based on the symptoms. Since a number of gene defects / mutations often associated with these diseases have recently been identified, it has unfortunately become a commonly held opinion that this disease is an immutable fate. However, when patients discuss the onset of the disease, it often becomes clear that there are clear links to psychological stress, dietary habits, medication use and preceding infections. The fact that the disease often first strikes between the ages of 20 and 40 is also revealing since this is often the period when the greatest stresses and strains are placed on an individual, both privately and professionally. Moreover, there is a statistical correlation between the occurrence of these diseases and the advancement of what we, perhaps erroneously, call civilisation. Such momentous shifts always come with significant new strains on humans by way of modern foods and additives, environmental toxins, hygiene measures etc. Ultimately, these bowel diseases involve dysfunctional regulation of the immune system, i.e. autoimmune or hyperimmune processes. That is why mainstream medicine mainly treats these diseases with long-term administration of anti-inflammatory (salicylic acid derivatives) medications, and medications which suppress the immune system (cortisone).

DMSO's various pharmacological properties – not least the anti-inflammatory, pain relief and regenerative effects – make it an obvious choice as a treatment for chronic inflammatory bowel disease. Its immune modulation effect may also play a part in stopping the disease from advancing or deteriorating further. A holistic assessment, taking a detailed case history, and a resulting individualised treatment plan can lead to a fundamental turnaround in the patient's condition.

Brain disorders (see also Arteriosclerosis, Infarction)

Broken bones See Sports injuries

Bronchitis See Respiratory tract infections

Bruises See Sports injuries

Burnout / bore-out

There is no need to discuss, as is done in research circles, whether these two conditions represent a distinct syndrome or whether they are a faddish figment of the imagination. As with any imbalance in the human body that has a clear psychological aspect, one should never be too hasty when judging what the main causes might be. We should, in such cases, surely be asking what came first: the chicken or the egg? Or to put it in another way, are psychological / neurological processes to blame or might it be due to other issues such as metabolic problems, deficiencies or immune system weaknesses? If you read a textbook on the illnesses of the organs – i.e. regarding pathology – you would be surprised to discover how many conditions that appear at first to be purely physical are actually attributable to the psyche. It is well known that patients who have an underactive thyroid (hypothyroidism) also exhibit symptoms of depression. Since everyone reacts in a unique way, it is sometimes the case that the other typical symptoms of this hormone deficiency are not particularly pronounced. Such a patient might then be incorrectly treated using dangerous antidepressants even though it would be easy and more effective to treat the root cause, the underactive thyroid. Patients suffering from vitamin B12 deficiency anaemia – a chronic blood formation problem that leads to a red blood cell deficiency – also face a similar scenario because they exhibit the symptoms of severe depression. Imagine how many pensioners have been given inappropriate neurological treatment as a result.

Now there are a host of less spectacular physiological problems that would often not be noticed in a blood test or a standard case history examination. Despite that, such issues lead, over a certain period of time, to entrenched chronic symptoms and diseases that we call burnout and bore-out syndrome. Generally speaking the patient perceives the condition in terms of reduced energy and performance. When the search for causes begins, it is not long before family and work are identified as being to blame. But what if we are barking up the wrong tree? What if we discover, by taking a more comprehensive and detailed case history, that the patient underwent a small, routine operation just before the complaints were noticed and that the surgical scar is still sensitive to changes in the weather or is disrupting an important meridian (neural pathway)? What if the patient suddenly remembers that long before the psychological symptoms developed they took antibiotics for seven days to treat an infection, and that they did not carry out an intestinal cleanse afterwards? What if we discover that mobile phone masts are causing extreme electrosmog at the workplace or that the new furnishing is giving off synthetic chemical emissions? What if the patient is suffering from long-term malnutrition and vitamin deficiency because of the poor quality food on offer at the canteen at work? What if an amalgam (mercury) filling was removed six months before the sudden drop in energy? This list, as I am sure you can imagine, could continue ad infinitum. The important point is that triggers that cause psychological symptoms down the line are physical and the symptoms they cause can be treated on the physical level – usually using very simple measures. It is obvious that an organism that is chronically overacidic, or that is vitamin deficient, or whose digestive system is deficient, will at some point not be able to perform as well as it used to. Viewed holistically, physical dysfunction naturally drags down the mind and the spirit, and burnout soon results. The converse can also be true of course – what is known as psychosomatic and somatoform disorders. Despite that, it is important not to over-hastily 'peg' patients, and burnout and bored-out patients in particular, as psychological cases.

What contribution can DMSO make? We know that this substance works as a regenerative agent. Regeneration means guiding physical functions back to their natural state. This takes place in a number of ways, including detoxification, and the regulation and modulation of enzymes. That is why DMSO can provide such important impulses in the early phases of burnout and bore-out treatment, impulses that also support any other measures taken. The decision regarding which other measures to take should be based on as detailed a case history and diagnosis as possible, and they should include improved nutrition, and measures to aid the musculoskeletal system, and sleep.

Treatment using DMSO: you can start treatment using initial doses of 0.05 to 0.1 gram of DMSO per kilogram of body weight once a day. DMSO can be taken as a 75% solution via the skin (preferably the legs) or drunk in a large glass of water. Infusions are also a suitable option. Depending on tolerance, you can then increase the daily dose to 0.3 to 0.5 gram per kilogram of body weight. You should take rest days and limit treatment to a period of two weeks at a time.

Burns See Wounds

Bursitis See Joint inflammation

Calcaneal spur (heel spur)

This condition involves the ossification of the tendon of the heel bone around the sole of the foot. This tissue damage can additionally lead to (chronic) inflammation, causing even more symptoms and pains. This is unfortunately the reality for many patients and the calcaneal spur has won a place as one of the most common orthopaedic diseases. For some patients the symptoms disappear after a certain time, for others the condition deteriorates until they can no longer walk. Discussing possible causes, such as the hard surfaces we walk on in the modern world or wearing shoes (neither of which evolution had in mind for us), is futile because we can hardly do anything to change these circumstances. Despite that I would recommend that anyone suffering from this or other foot conditions walk barefoot whenever they can. The condition may worsen initially as you take a few days to adjust but this simple measure, which is free of charge, can quickly lead to the relief of movement pains and to a brand new feeling of physical well-being and balance.

As a pain reliever and anti-inflammatory agent, DMSO is an effective treatment for heel spurs. It is one of many musculoskeletal conditions that usually respond quickly to this kind of treatment, bringing great relief for patients. It brings with it the risk that patients, delighted that they can walk without pain once more, put too much strain on the area too soon. The tissue must be allowed time to regenerate after the pain has disappeared. For that to happen, the inflammation must subside and the toxic substances that have accumulated in that area over a long period of time must be broken down and eliminated. The improved nutritional status of the tendon and bone, brought about by the DMSO, must be put to use for repair purposes. A 70 to 80% DMSO solution is applied liberally to the sole of the foot and all around the ankle. Once the first application has been absorbed by the skin, immediately apply a second and third dose in the same way. Over the following few weeks, the treatment should be repeated daily up to twice a day to ensure a long-term cure. In very persistent cases you can resort to using a highly effective mixture of diclofenac in DMSO (e.g. Voltaren® gel). However, diclofenac should be used cautiously. This medication must be handled carefully and responsibly because of contraindications (chronic inflammatory bowel diseases, asthma, etc.), side effects and drug interactions. The drug also causes a very specific water cycle problem. The German Wikipedia entry on diclofenac states: '70% of diclofenac leaves the human body unaltered. About 90 tonnes of this medication are used in Germany each year, causing 63 tonnes of it to be flushed via the urine into the water cycle. Since the wastewater treatment plants are not designed to process it, medications and their residues make their way almost unhindered via the surface water back to our drinking-water. In India in the 1990s, diclofenac treatment for cattle unexpectedly caused a drastic reduction in the vulture population, making it necessary to implement conservation measures. The birds were taking in the medication via the carcasses of animals. The sick vultures first exhibited symptoms resembling gout, before ultimately dying of kidney failure. The use of diclofenac in veterinary medicine has been outlawed in India since 2005.'

Unfortunately, the relaxation of diclofenac's 'prescription-only' status has led to the inflationary use of the substance, which was excessive even when it required a doctor's signature (although from the perspective of the pharmaceutical companies this is the whole point of relaxing the regulations).

But to return to the heel spur: buy a cheap pain relief gel containing diclofenac at your local pharmacy and mix the desired quantity in a glass with DMSO so that you have a 1:1 liquid mixture of both ingredients. Apply this to the painful area of the foot once and leave it for as long as possible to be absorbed. This method should only be repeated once every three to four days at the most. It can cause serious damage to the skin if applied more often.

Case: Ms F. S., 51 years old, had been suffering from a chronic, deteriorating heel spur for four years. Her gait and posture had become extremely unbalanced and she had tried a number of mainstream medical treatments to no avail. I recommended that she try the approach described above, for which she bought a spray bottle containing a 75% DMSO solution in water. The pains reduced significantly after only two applications (she sprayed the whole of her foot) and she regained the ability to do a number of things that she had long grown accustomed to missing. She continued to administer DMSO once every day over the following weeks. Seeing the constant improvement, she continued to take the time to carry out the self-treatment and stayed motivated.

Cancer

It is easy to find statistics on the internet that reveal how poor the recovery rates for cancer are, even today, when the disease is treated with chemotherapy, operations and radiation. These are not statistics collated by amateurs or 'professional sceptics', but are officially documented and taken from scientific and medical statistical surveys. We are familiar with the fairy tales which speak of the purported advancements in treatment using new radiation methods or chemically modified drugs; these tales have circulated for at least fifty years. All too often these efforts, which devour unbelievable sums of public and private research funding (our money, in part), serve only to increase the reputation of individual research institutions and the professors who work there, all of whom seek international recognition. As part of that work, legions of junior researchers 'serve' in the laboratories, most of whom are probably completely unaware that their work, when viewed from afar, is reminiscent of poor Don Quixote's futile battles. We already know how to repair dysfunctional cell metabolism and how to rectify the mutated growth patterns that arise as a result, which means that we could be conducting far more research on targeted, appropriate (natural) substances. Of course, this approach does not come with the promise of substantial profits from new, patentable products which the powerful pharmaceutical giants push onto the 'health market' (or should we say the 'disease market') via the medical fraternity. And so we are left to continue to yearn for a world in which everyone aspires to an 'open source mentality' for the good of **all** patients. Or we can take matters into our own hands!

Even medical researchers working in the public sector have, in meta-analytical studies, repeatedly demonstrated that the five-year survival rate following mainstream medical treatment alone is, on average, still in the low single figures. However, a blind belief in doctors that is firmly anchored in the collective subconscious means that we continue to cling to a warped image of reality. Having been diagnosed with cancer, most patients see their only chance for survival in what is presented to them by the hospital as a progressive and promising solution. That is a good business model, no doubt. But even the much-loved Apotheken Umschau (a German medical magazine for lay people) recently published a critical report on the severe long-term negative side effects of mainstream cancer treatments and questioned the soundness of the standard approach.

Mutated cells – that is what we are dealing with in cancer cases – no longer do what they are supposed to be doing according to the genes. I do not intend to take sides with any theory regarding the cause of such cell mutations here. However, we can be sure that cancer does not appear from nowhere. Some people rattle on adamantly about natural radioactivity or cosmic radiation (which might be said to 'appear from nowhere') that can cause cell mutations. But evolution has taken these earthly conditions into consideration and has equipped all living creatures with a corresponding level of immunity. This kind of cell mutation occurs in the body a number of times per week on average, but not everyone becomes ill with cancer. Normally the cells themselves or the immune cells responsible know when radiation has caused cell damage. The mitochondria then initiate a self-destruction programme or the phagocytes and killer cells quickly take care of the matter. However, it appears that adverse metabolic processes or (viral) infections are responsible for the formation of cancer cells far more often than physical causes such as the above. With adverse metabolic processes, cancer would have to be categorised as a disease of civilisation (overeating, overacidification, etc.) while in the case of (viral) infections, cancer would have to be categorised as an immune system deficiency. Since a strong immune system is particularly dependent on appropriate nutrition, exercise, sunlight, positive emotions etc., we can confidently assume that cancer is the aggregation of chronic tissue imbalances. Defined generally in this way, it fits in with a large number of alternative and mainstream theories on the cause of malignant diseases. Unfortunately the term 'malignant' gives the impression that these rampant cells have decided to deliberately cause us problems. As Otto Warburg (doctor and biochemist, Nobel Prize for Medicine, 1931) hypothesised, however, we can assume that individual cells that switch their metabolism to an anaerobic process of energy production are only following a self-preservation instinct. In a manner of speaking, one could even say that these cancer cells 'think' that it is their surroundings (the matrix) and not themselves that is 'malignant' (i.e. overacidic or oxygen-poor).

I will not go into this subject in more detail here. It is sufficient to point briefly to the fact that cancer often (or always) has its origins in dietary habits, the toxic load in the body, and other physical states unfavourable to health. We can logically draw the conclusion that such a disease should be treated using only measures that help to reduce the toxic load and support the immune system. Can you think of any arguments in favour of using treatments such as chemotherapy and radiation that increase the toxic load and suppress the immune system?

The problem is that many patients are keen to use alternative cancer treatments but do not reject mainstream medical options outright. One obvious reason for this is the scare tactics used by doctors to make their patients compliant in their helpless state. One patient suffering from bladder cancer told me that his previous doctor had given him the following warning: 'If you don't have an operation and start radiation treatment at once, you'll croak like a dog before Christmas!' The patient told me this smiling with satisfaction the following February having refused further treatment from that physician.

While ever increasing sums of money are being pumped into 'approved' cancer research with no corresponding improvement in results, we read countless convincing reports by recovered cancer patients who used very simple, often extremely cheap medications. Among them are reports of cures for breast cancer, colon cancer, pancreatic cancer, stomach cancer, lung cancer, bone cancer, lymph gland cancer, skin cancer and many others. The (self-) treatment programmes used always involve more than one element. Alongside the administration of highly effective substances such as DMSO, MMS, lactic acid, oxidants, fruit kernels, alkalines, vitamins and others, many patients report making changes to their diet, lifestyles, work and place of residence, as well as making other important life decisions. Here too it is obvious that we encourage a holistic approach to healing.

DMSO can be used on its own or it can be used in combination with other substances to treat cancer. The regenerative and cell-protection effects of DMSO shine through most clearly in the way the patient's general condition quickly stabilises, and in the reduction of fatigue symptoms. The immune system is strengthened and detoxification processes are supported. DMSO optimises the transportation of selective oxidants (MMS, etc.) and cell-repairers (right-turning lactic acid, procaine, etc.) through the body. Doses and application methods can be adjusted to suit each individual's situation and condition, following the suggestions made in Chapter 2. When we supervise cancer patients it always becomes particularly clear to us how important it is to regard the development of the disease as a providential path. It is also striking how much the various influencing factors pull the patient in various directions, making their treatment decisions even more difficult.

The following example illustrates this clearly. A young man (37 years old), accompanied by his parents, sought my advice towards the end of November 2011 having undergone mainstream medical treatment for a pancreatic tumour for some months. He had had various chemotherapy treatments and had been operated on twice, only to establish that the growing tumour could not be removed. He regarded his visit to my practice as a last-ditch effort because he had been told that he had no hope of a recovery. He had undergone the latest operation just three days earlier. As you would expect, he was weak and debilitated, particularly so since he had been suffering from a fatigue disorder before the cancer developed and he was now suffering from pronounced tumour anaemia. Since he lived more than 300km away from my clinic we arranged to have him remain in the area for a week, during which time he would come to the clinic twice a day. He was to start a combined MMS and DMSO treatment as soon as possible. We gave him the first two doses of these substances immediately as a solution to drink. In addition, we stabilised his condition through acupuncture treatment on general energy points, sent a blood test to the laboratory, and I cleared the disturbance fields on the fresh scars on his abdomen using a DMSO–procaine solution. Within half an hour he reported that the pains were abating and that he was no longer shivering. The tension in the abdominal wall disappeared and some colour had returned to his face. The next morning the patient spoke of horrendous hotel beds and diarrhoea – the first sign of MMS detoxification. Sleep had not been restorative and the abdominal wall was painful again. The blood counts were at the same levels as those taken at the hospital. We increased the dose of DMSO and MMS taken orally, and also started administering the oxidative substance as an infusion. In the meantime the patient was able to prepare his own doses of the medication and reported gratifying progress from day to day. I used the time in the clinic for long conversations to stabilise him emotionally. Even then it often appeared that he was reluctant to turn his back completely on Chemo & Co., despite the bad experience he had had with it overall. His thoughts were never clear and rational even though the facts up to that point were unambiguous, a process that cannot be comprehended; a characteristic that has been inherent in humans from the earliest stages of our development. Also typical was the way he put forward a number of 'good arguments' for thinking in this way. The supervising oncologist back home was a friend of the family. The cancer clinic had told him he could take part in a study of a 'brand new, highly targeted' treatment. But that was conditional upon him continuing with the regular chemotherapy treatment that he had started. If he did this, he would enjoy the privilege of special and far more thorough diagnosis methods than previously. And so on. And so on.

I explained my point of view to him and he returned home at the end of the week with improved blood counts, physical improvements and a sense of hope. We stayed in touch with weekly phone consultations and he continued with the treatment measures we had started. He saw constant improvements. Unfortunately he soon wanted to stop taking the DMSO, feeling that the smell was too much of a burden on the family. He also mentioned the 'progress' made regarding his application to be accepted onto the cancer study, which he was becoming increasingly excited about. Even though he and his father were both unambiguous in their descriptions of the days of staggering suffering brought on by each new dose of his oncologist's chemical cocktail, he could not resist the 'promise' and he put up with the setbacks. One step forward, two steps back. When the study began he was required to stop taking all other medications: that was a fundamental condition. Our telephone conversations then also became increasingly irregular.

At the time, I felt that alternative medicine had lost him by then – or the other way around! Once or twice he mentioned the way the study was being conducted at the cancer clinic, which was to my mind highly questionable. A few weeks after the introduction of the new substance (or a placebo? – after all, it was a double-blind trial) he wanted to arrange an appointment to see me again. The way he discussed his participation in the study was sobering and he could not identify any advantage from taking part. The first reports came in of companions in the clinical trial who had died of their pancreatic tumours. He had, once again, been told that there was nothing that could be done for him. The comprehensive diagnostic measures had not shown any improvements over the weeks of treatment at the cancer clinic. On that day the patient, now extremely weakened and physically unstable again, asked me once more whether he should continue with the chemotherapy.

A few weeks later he called me, speaking very faintly, apologising that he had not called for such a long time and asking whether he could restart treatment with me. Since he felt he was no longer able to travel I promised to look for a health practitioner in his area who was proficient in the appropriate methods. When I called two days later to give him the address, his wife told me that he had died the previous day. She thanked me sincerely for the extra few months of progress and hope that her husband had received through my treatment.

There is a wide range of ways in which DMSO can be combined with other effective anti-cancer medications. One in particular – haematoxylin – is discussed here. Morton Walker[19] describes the use of this substance as a cancer treatment based on a case example of a patient. Joe Floyd, then 56 years old and a manager at the Exxon Oil company, in April 1974 suffered from a bleeding rectal carcinoma. This form of adenocarcinoma is highly malignant, grows quickly and is acutely life-threatening. The patient suffered from constipation, severe pain, bleeding, fever, night sweats, weakness, and he was losing weight quickly. At the time of the diagnosis, Joe Floyd already had metastases in the neighbouring lymph nodes and in the liver. The company physician sent him to a colon surgeon in Houston, who removed 33cm of his colon as well as the affected lymph nodes. The doctor told Joe Floyd to start the scheduled chemotherapy treatment. The doctor revealed that his wife had also fallen ill with the same condition around the same time and that she would be starting the same treatment programme following her operation. However, Joe Floyd refused this conventional treatment because he remembered a report he had seen on television two years previously. The report had featured an alternative cancer treatment offered by Dr Elliot Tucker, who also practiced in Houston. Tucker used a mixture of

DMSO and haematoxylin (a natural dye, see Chapter 2.5.3), which he had discovered was a highly effective treatment for cancer. Joe Floyd wanted to know more about this method. After some serious persuasion, Dr Tucker agreed to treat the patient on the latter's responsibility. Six weeks later the surgeon's wife, who had decided to take the standard chemotherapy treatment, died. But Joe Floyd was back at his desk in the Exxon offices and continued to receive an infusion every other day at Tucker's clinic. He did not suffer any nausea whatsoever, or any other symptoms associated with chemotherapy. After 18 months, Tucker finally discharged him, saying he was completely cured. His CEA marker was below the normal value. In May 1989, Morton Walker spoke to Joe Floyd, now 71 years of age, who was enjoying excellent health and had opened a health food shop, which was a great source of satisfaction for him in his retirement.

Based on further experiences Dr Tucker shows that the DMSO–haematoxylin mixture can be used with particular success to treat large-cell lymphoma. It can be used to treat both humans and animals. You will find relevant examples of its use in Morton Walker's book.

The stories of these patients demonstrate that DMSO should be given an important place in alternative cancer treatment. DMSO combined with other substances (right-turning lactic acid, DCA, lipoic acid, MMS, etc.), together with diet and lifestyle changes, provides far more hope of a cure than anything the mainstream medical system can offer. Of primary importance here are clear decisions by the patient in favour of natural methods of treatment that are geared towards strengthening (not weakening!) the body's own powers of self-healing. DMSO is ideally suited for this, as you can imagine having read about its pharmacological properties. Depending on the specific form of the disease, DMSO can be administered via the skin, taken as a drink solution, or via infusion. The dose depends on individual circumstances and the progression of the disease (see Chapter 2).

Carcinomas See Cancer

Cataract See Eye diseases

Chemotherapy side effects (see also Chronic fatigue syndrome)
Chemotherapy medications often have a cytostatic effect, i.e. they inhibit cell growth and cell division, and suppress the immune system. The

cytostatic damage is most noticeable in cells that have a naturally high division and metabolic rate. These include (along with the tumour cells themselves) gastrointestinal epithelial cells and bone marrow cells that are responsible for the formation of new red and white blood cells. This is why patients suffer from serious gastrointestinal problems and anaemia (blood cell deficiency) during / after chemotherapy treatment. This, in turn, leads to chronic fatigue, exhaustion and, above all, oxygen defiency – establishing a vicious circle. There is also an immune vulnerability because of a deficiency of white blood cells (cells of the immune system). This can lead to increased infections, fungal diseases etc. All these and other symptoms are summarised under the term 'chronic fatigue syndrome'. DMSO use can be very effective in just the same way that it supports regeneration and accelerates recovery following operations or infections. Anyone who has decided to undergo conventional medical treatment for cancer (medications or radiation) can stabilise their condition by taking DMSO both before and after treatment. The best way to do this is to take the recommended doses given in Chapter 2 in the form of aqueous solutions via the skin or as a drink or an infusion. The most appropriate administration method will depend on individual circumstances. In cases of severe gastrointestinal problems it may be better to start with external applications via the skin or with infusions before transferring to a drink solution at gradually increasing doses.

Chilblains

DMSO protects cells from frost – that was the original medicinal use discovered by Dr Stanley Jacob. That has no practical benefits for us in winter because no one is likely to take DMSO continuously simply to prevent potential damage by frost. When the tissue at exposed areas of the body such as the fingers, ears, chin, cheeks and toes has been damaged by cold, the affected areas of skin become very red, accompanied by hardening, and a painful, itching swelling. Fortunately, DMSO can be applied as a regenerative substance that accelerates the healing of the inflammatory reaction. Apply an aqueous DMSO solution liberally to the chilblains (external application). A 50 to 75% preparation should be used, depending on which area of the body is affected. Lower doses are used on the face while higher doses can be used on the fingers and toes. Last winter I used this method to cure some very unpleasant chilblains on our daughter's cheeks and chin. Her face had not felt cold while she was sledging but the ice-cold airflow had bitten into the exposed areas of skin. You might consider treating in advance areas typically affected by cold if you intend to take part in activities such as winter sports that involve potentially dangerous exposure to frost and cold air.

Child psychosis See Developmental disorders in children

Chronic fatigue syndrome

The exact definition of this term is constantly under discussion. Exhaustion can arise as a stand-alone disease or in connection with other underlying illnesses. States of chronic exhaustion that include both subjectively perceived symptoms and objectively measureable symptoms such as anaemia or other deficiencies are common elements of the following diseases: cancer, multiple sclerosis, chronic infections, chronic heart and lung diseases, rheumatism, AIDS, Crohn's disease, ankylosing spondylitis, fibromyalgia, etc. Chronic states of exhaustion can also develop independently of any underlying disease. Symptoms can include constantly irritated lymph nodes, sore throat, joint and muscle pains, concentration problems, headaches, reduced energy, and sleep disorders. Even if no obvious cause can be identified, in the field of alternative medicine we work on the assumption that many of the patients who suffer from chronic fatigue are suffering chronic viral, bacterial or parasite infections. Other considerations are chronically disturbed intestinal flora, toxic loads, metabolic problems, and interference fields.

Chronic fatigue is a condition that should be taken seriously, requiring a very detailed case history to be taken and a precise diagnosis to be made. DMSO can be a very useful treatment because the substance's various complementary properties work on different levels in the body to regulate physical processes. Because of the intense suffering that has led most patients to seek out a health practitioner, DMSO infusions are particularly suitable as a 'first aid' measure that can have a quick effect. Other basic treatment options include special cleansing, detoxification and deacidification measures.

One female patient (38 years old), who does not want to be named, had been suffering from a (subjectively perceived) lack of energy for a long time. She also had constantly irritated / swollen lymph nodes and was battling insomnia. In addition, she had a host of other complaints that limited her life, including digestive problems, shivering / sweating and muscle pains. The woman was in such a bad state that she had begun to assume that her illness was psychological in origin. A comprehensive clinical examination finally raised suspicions that a reactivated chronic EBV infection (Epstein–Barr Virus) might be causing the problems. That in itself is not uncommon since almost 100% of the over-40s are infected with it. This virus, also known as human herpesvirus 4, remains in the body for life after it is first contracted early on in life ('kissing disease' or 'student's disease'). Only in very few cases is the virus reactivated, resulting in the corresponding symptoms. This can occur during (temporary) phases of immune system weakness, for example. The German Wikipedia entry on the Epstein–Barr Virus (accessed 20/4/2012) states: 'Recently, it is increasingly suspected that EBV is linked to a range of autoimmune diseases such as multiple sclerosis, systemic lupus erythematosus and rheumatoid arthritis. [...] It is also thought that there is a link between the virus and chronic fatigue syndrome (according to research at Berlin's Charité) and encephalitis lethargica.'

On my recommendation the patient took increasing doses of MMS and DMSO and, after a few days, reported that she had found a new lease of life. Also using other small supporting measures the symptoms disappeared or abated gradually. She was sleeping well, felt able to cope with her work and private life and the swollen lymph nodes had reduced significantly. When I saw her two weeks later she looked as if many years had rolled away from her.

Circulatory disorders

Circulatory disorders have far-reaching effects that contribute to the development of a number of chronic conditions. At the root of all the diseases that belong to this category lies an oxygen and nutrient deficiency and an accumulation of waste (metabolic end products) in the affected parts of the body. We speak of angina pectoris when the coronary blood vessel does not allow sufficient blood through for the supply and elimination of substances to and from the heart muscle. Or we speak of peripheral artery occlusive disease (PAOD) when the arteries in the legs do not allow sufficient blood through to supply the muscles in that area of the body. That forces the patient to sit down after walking a short distance, allowing the muscles to recover and the pain to abate. Our first priority on encountering these disorders is to ensure an unrestricted (or as close to that as possible) supply of oxygen-rich, arterial blood to all the tissues in the body. However, in some cases the pathological process may only creep in gradually without any dramatic symptoms such as severe chest pains or significant restriction in natural movement. A number of holistic doctors and alternative health practitioners have pointed out in countless books that some severe chronic diseases, including cancer, are ultimately caused by oxygen and / or nutrient deficiency, as well as by the gradual accumulation of waste products / toxins when not eliminated efficiently in the long term. The main reason for this is always circulation problems. Body tissue in areas of the body that need exceptionally high levels of blood react particularly sensitively to even the slightest disturbance to the supply and elimination of substances. These include the kidneys, the central nervous system (brain and spinal cord), the liver, the heart, and the lungs.

The same is true for areas of the body that naturally only receive very little nutrition or that are supplied only through diffusion processes. These include the joints and their layers of cartilage. That can result in the patient developing very common disorders such as kidney damage, memory problems / dizziness, liver damage accompanied by digestive problems, angina pectoris, breathlessness and arthrosis. These pathological processes have the greatest impact on the capillary bed, the area of the smallest of all the blood vessels (capillaries). This is where all the substances are exchanged and these processes are dependent on the permeability of the capillaries in both directions. What I mean by that is that there is unhindered movement in the direction of the blood flow as well as in the 'sideways' movement of diffusion through the walls of the capillaries. Only in this way can nutrients be transported into the tissue and waste be transported out. The lymph flow, which plays an important part in detoxification, is also passively regulated here.

So what are the causes of circulation problems? To find the answer we need to look at the 'pipelines' or the blood vessels themselves, and the 'liquid organ', the blood that flows through them. When their diameter is reduced the blood vessels allow less blood to flow through them. That can be caused by elevated tonus (tension) in the musculature of the vessel wall, or by waste deposits. In both instances we would be able to diagnose elevated blood pressure because a narrowing of the pathways leads to an increase in pressure. You will be familiar with that if you have read the instructions regarding the use of your garden hose nozzle. With regard to the substance flowing in the vessels, it is only logical that an increase in viscosity (a thickening of the liquid) will result in a reduced flow rate. Blood consists of a liquid solution (water with electrolytes, proteins, glucose, gasses etc.) and solid constituent elements that swim in it. These solid elements are mainly blood cells (red and white blood cells). If the proportion of the liquid solution is reduced and the influence of the blood cells on the fluidity is thereby increased, the blood flows at a slower rate as a result. One cause of such changes to viscosity is lack of water, other causes include blood formation problems (originating in the bone marrow), and coagulation problems.

If you now review all the listed causes of circulatory problems and compare them to the pharmacological properties of DMSO, it will be clear that this substance will make a comprehensive contribution to improving circulation. DMSO inhibits blood coagulation, expands the blood vessels, reduces muscle tension, prevents / reduces deposits and flushes out the build-up of liquids in the tissue that limits the exchange processes in the capillary bed. Incredible, isn't it? All this can usually be achieved with the regular or intermittent administration of 0.05 to 0.2 grams of DMSO per kilogram of body weight once a day. Apply the appropriate quantity of DMSO solution to the skin, drink the DMSO in a heavily diluted mixture, or administer as an infusion solution. All three methods are explained in detail in Chapter 2.

Colds See Respiratory tract infections

Colitis See Bowel diseases

Complex regional pain syndrome

This condition, with its slightly unusual and complicated-sounding name, occurs more often than you might think. Other names used to describe this condition include reflex sympathetic dystrophy, Sudeck's atrophy, and reflex neurovascular dystrophy. The word 'dystrophy' is very helpful; it indicates the degeneration of tissue due to disease or malnutrition. The disease develops as a result of some kind of external influence: falls (e.g. fractured bones), operations (e.g. carpal tunnel, ankle) or infections (e.g. bacterial inflammations in open wounds). The condition causes pain, fluid retention, skin problems, dysfunction in certain parts of the body, and circulation problems in the arms or the legs. Statistically, complex regional pain syndrome occurs most often after fracturing the bones of the forearm, for example in cycling accidents. The injury appears to heal well initially, but in some people the symptoms described above subsequently develop. This usually leads to a long story of suffering with little chance of a cure. Patients often say such things as: 'No one can tell me what it is', or 'They don't do anything other than give me painkillers ... and it's getting worse', or 'If only I hadn't agreed to that operation.' The exact causes and the pathology of the genesis of these severe complications are not fully understood. Despite that, alternative methods such as neural therapy, acupuncture and DMSO offer significantly better results than treating the symptoms using standard painkillers or cortisone. DMSO has a multipronged effect, improving the supply and detoxification processes to and from the affected area. Other important effects include the reduction of swelling, pain relief, and improvement in circulation.

In cases of complex regional pain syndrome, DMSO is mainly used locally, externally. An aqueous solution of the substance is applied liberally to the affected area. Since it is usually the (fore-)arms and (lower) legs that are affected, and since the pains are usually severe, higher concentrations should be used. The 65 to 80% DMSO solution is best applied intensively all around the affected area using a brush. Expect to see a reduction in symptoms after the first application. However, the treatment should be continued over a long period of time. After applying the DMSO it will probably be necessary to treat and soothe the main areas affected and damaged by the disease with aloe vera preparations (which should be as pure as possible). In severe cases you might in the early phases of treatment want to consider taking DMSO orally or intravenously at the same time as the external application. The appropriate dose is based on body weight, as described in Chapter 2.

Concentration problems See Developmental disorders in children

Cortisone therapy

Cortisone therapy is of course not a disease itself, but a treatment often used for a number of (chronic) illnesses. Cortisone is usually administered externally (creams, ointments) and internally in tablet form. The application of sprays and nebulisers to treat respiratory diseases can also be regarded as topical administrations in a certain sense ('inner surface'). DMSO amplifies the effect of a number of other medications significantly, and when cortisone is combined with DMSO its effect can be multiplied by a factor of between 10 and 1000 because of the improved penetration of biological membranes.

This effect is widely used in veterinary medicine. The Dexamethason in DMSO® preparation by CP-Pharma is understandably popular with vets and is used externally to treat joint diseases, injuries, inflamed tendons, etc. However, the real advantage of mixtures of cortisone and DMSO is that it allows the quantity of cortisone administered to be reduced since its efficacy is increased. This is very important. You probably know that cortisone can have serious side effects even when only taken over short periods of time. The risk of suppressing the body's own production of adrenocortical hormones rises sharply when doses higher than 20mg of cortisol equivalent are taken for more than 7 days (known as the 'Cushing threshold').

By taking DMSO at the same time, the cortisone dose can in many cases be adjusted downwards, which is a significant relief for patients. Caution: systemically administered cortisone should not be suddenly discontinued. It takes experience and a good instinct to adjust and set doses. If you have questions regarding changing the dose of internal cortisone administration when combining it with DMSO, you should consult a specialist.

I generally advise against taking any pharmaceutical cortisone medication no matter what claims they might make regarding it being 'side effect-free'. This includes creams, sprays and tinctures for local application, not to mention tablets. Experience has shown, as any accredited and respected alternative medicine practitioner will tell you, that even a single application of cortisone can cause long-term structural and vegetative damage which is difficult to control.

Crohn's disease See Bowel diseases

Dementia See Neurodegenerative diseases

Developmental disorders in children

DMSO can help in almost all problems related to the development of children. There is also evidence to suggest that these findings are also applicable to adults. Dr Morton Walker[19] provides a useful summary of this topic in the chapter entitled 'DMSO Therapy for Mental Disabilities', but repeatedly emphasises that motor skills impairments, learning difficulties and mental abnormalities (in infancy) all belong to the same group. When used to treat such conditions, the universal balancing effect of DMSO comes to the fore, bringing about a measurable normalisation of a number of physiological processes. This is evident even when treating irreversible conditions such as trisomy 21 (see Down's syndrome). Young patients (and older ones) with learning difficulties, low intelligence, ADHD, anxiety disorders, epilepsy, nervousness, dyscalculia, dyslexia, exhaustion, and concentration problems all benefit even more when certain amino acids that support neurotransmitter balance in the brain are administered in combination with DMSO. These were the findings of one research project that resulted in the introduction in South America of ready-to-use ampule preparations containing this mixture. Amino acids such as gamma aminobutyric acid, N-acetylglutamate and others are mixed with DMSO. The simultaneous administration of these protein building blocks and DMSO promotes the development of brain functions and activity because the DMSO carries the amino acids into the central nervous system.

A research project in Chile led by Dr Carlos Nassar involved the treatment of 44 schoolchildren with learning and developmental problems and who exhibited low mental capacity. The case histories of the children included a number of indications that they were late learning to walk, talk, and master psychomotor skills. They were aggressive for no reason, rebellious, irritable, or had epileptic episodes. Their IQ levels were tested before treatment began and again after three, six and ten months of DMSO administration. The advancements in mental capacity ascertained by Dr Nasser were exceptional. Even though a number of other treatment methods had previously only brought extremely limited results if any at all, more than 70% of the children involved in the study now exhibited positive responses with increased learning ability after only a relatively short period of time. They achieved higher IQ values, significantly quicker progress in basic skills, better overall intellectual capacities, clear development in their reading, writing and mathematical abilities, improved movement coordination and dexterity, and fewer behavioural problems.

This astonishing therapeutic success has been reproduced in other research projects, for example in a study involving fifty children between the ages of 5 and 15 who all had speech and language disorders. After six months of treatment using the DMSO and amino acid combination, all the children exhibited remarkable development. The neuropsychiatrist Dr Azael Paz attributes this to a stimulation of the oxidative energy metabolism in the brain. The researchers summarised the results as follows (see Morton Walker,[19] pp. 172–3):

- continuous development of the child's ability to experience greater awareness
- changes and progress in the child's moral attitude
- unfolding of the personality
- dawning of self-criticism
- satisfaction in establishing their own personal identity

Referring to the initial symptoms observed in the children, they summed up the improvements as follows:

- disappearance of mental lethargy
- evidence of sensorial reactions
- disappearance of automatic movements (twitches, ticks)
- disappearance of inertia, passivity and negativity
- growing interest and initiative in tasks and activities
- improvements in physiognomic expression and spoken language
- lucid activity, group contact, and disappearance of unprovoked aggressiveness
- losing shyness, developing self-esteem
- successful training to carry out chores, shopping, etc.
- learning to read, write and do their homework

Unfortunately, the ampules containing the DMSO and amino acid mixture are not available in Europe. Instead, you can use DMSO on its own or DMSO in combination with an appropriate nutritional therapy approach. Combinations of DMSO with nutritional supplements rich in amino acids such as cereal grasses (barley grass powder) are also suitable alternatives. However, it is important that you consider at what time of day these nutrients are best processed and absorbed by the body after eating. The third option is to buy the individual amino acids contained in the South American preparations (Akron®, Merinex®) and to mix them yourself. In my experience it is good to supplement these ingredients with galactose. Galactose is a carbohydrate present in breast milk that helps in particular by naturally supporting the rapid development of the brain in the first months of life.

Dog bites

The information presented in this section is also applicable to similar injuries from bites by other animals. I have personally had a very good experience of treating a dog bite using DMSO. Our ten-year-old daughter was bitten on the wrist by an unfamiliar dog while she was playing. The dog was actually quite friendly and only wanted to 'keep her' for himself. The dog owner became very agitated and my daughter was in shock. Luckily there was a bottle of a 75% DMSO solution at hand because the dog owner is a patient of mine who had invited us to have dinner with his family. I asked for the DMSO and dabbed some onto the bite wound, which had quickly become red and swollen. Along with giving all involved a sense of reassurance, the DMSO brought about the disappearance of the swelling and the pain within a few minutes. The wounds had healed completely by the following day.

Down's syndrome (see also Developmental disorders in children)

This genetic disorder, also known as trisomy 21, occurs in about 1 in 600 newborn babies (based on all live births). The motor (movement) and cognitive (language, stimulus processing) skills of children born with the condition develop at about half the usual pace in the first few years. Noticeable physical characteristics include slanted eyes, extra space between the big toe and the small toes, and a protruding tongue. Since those affected are, generally speaking, suffering from a developmental disorder we can expect DMSO to have an extremely positive effect both on the physical (e.g. muscle weakness) and on the mental disabilities. That is why the suggestions made here, as well as those made in the 'Developmental disorders in children' section, are applicable to other conditions involving developmental delays in children. These include isolated muscle weakness (muscle dystrophies, floppy infant), mental disabilities, hyperkinesia / hyperactivity, attention deficit disorders, dyslexia and dyscalculia, psychoses and anxiety in childhood years. It is often advisable in such cases to combine DMSO with concentrated amino acids and / or galactose. Galactose is a carbohydrate present in breast milk and which helps in particular by supporting the rapid development of the brain in the first months of life. It is therefore certainly worth experimenting with such mixtures to find the best possible support for affected children. It is worth reading the following case report documented by Dr Morton Walker:[19]

The Clarks were given a conclusive diagnosis for their daughter Melody when she was six months old – Down's syndrome. They were told that Melody's mental capacities would, in all likelihood, never develop past those of a six-year-old child. When she was eleven months old she began a DMSO treatment programme under the guidance of

Dr Stanley Jacob. At that time she was unable to turn herself from her back onto her stomach and her legs were still as limp as those of a rag doll. She could not focus her eyes at all and could hardly see. From that point onwards Melody was regularly given her dose of DMSO and by the time she was eight, she had developed from being a severely disabled child to being unusually highly developed. She ran, did somersaults and bounced on her trampoline. She was in second grade at school and excelled at arithmetic. Melody understood maths problems and was a good reader and talker. She attended Sunday school with the other children and was able to enjoy the 1980 summer camp with them. It is also important to note that she was very popular among her classmates. She had very good social skills. It was not just her mental development that was remarkable but also the physical changes in her were surprising. Her facial features changed. Her dentist, Dr David K. Priebe, who had been treating her over the years confirmed that the palatal roof, tongue size and tooth interspaces were now within the normal range. He also remarked that Melody coped with the stress of dental treatment just as well as children without trisomy 21. The girl was held in high esteem by her peers because of her personal merits and the teachers agreed that Melody had made huge leaps forward in all areas of her academic, social and physical development. Melody's mother wants DMSO to be available to all those affected, giving hope to parents like her. Scientists, however, still do not understand how DMSO brought about the changes in Melody and in other children with Down's syndrome. What is undeniable, however, is that DMSO worked these changes. Dr Jacob has treated hundreds of children with trisomy 21. Another research project carried out by Spanish doctors in 1982 has confirmed that children with Down's syndrome exhibit positive social developments when given DMSO treatment.

Drug addiction See Withdrawal symptoms

Dyslexia / dyscalculia and other impairments to higher cortical functions See Developmental disorders in children

Dystrophy / Sudeck's atrophy See Complex regional pain syndrome

Ear infections

A distinction is made between inflammations of the ear canal (*Otitis externa*) and acute or chronic inflammations of the middle ear (*Otitis media*). Whereas in the past it was common to prescribe systemic anti-biotics to children suffering from inflammation of the middle ear, today it is more common to follow the 'wait-and-see' strategy. Doctors now usually treat patients using only the painkiller ibuprofen, which also has an anti-inflammatory effect. For many years oral antibiotics were used – an approach that takes a great toll on children's bodies in partic-ular (damaging the intestinal flora).The argument used in support of that approach was that without it there was the risk of suffering serious complications from inflammation of the middle ear, and the fact that it was impossible to administer the antibiotic using ear drops. That would have required a medication that was able to pass through the eardrum, which separates the outer and middle ear.

This state of affairs has changed now that we are familiar with DMSO's amazing properties. There is still a risk of severe complications if the inflammation of the middle ear gets out of control and that is why it is important to carefully observe the development of the condition. DMSO does, however, solve the problem of how to transport the antibiotic substance through the eardrum. Applying correspondingly small doses of this kind of medication locally means that a number of side effects can be avoided. We can treat inflammations of the middle ear 'from the outside' using a mixture of DMSO and antibiotic ear drops. A commer-cial product based on this principle is apparently being tested at the moment. Those who find this approach too mainstream and who want to avoid using antibiotics altogether can use DMSO alone or in combi-nation with the alternative bactericides MMS or hydrogen peroxide, again in the form of an ear drop. A 40% DMSO solution is the most ap-propriate choice for this kind of application. Lying on one side, put 2 to 3 drops of this into the ear canal. A few drops of an MMS solution (2 drops of activated MMS in 10ml water) or a 1 to 3% hydrogen peroxide solution can be put in the ear immediately before or after. To disinfect injuries to the eardrum, 1 to 3% hydrogen peroxide can be used.

Case: one of my patients who had bought some DMSO for oral admin-istration told me one day that he had been treating his son, who suffered from recurring inflammations of the middle ear, with DMSO, admin-istering it when the son was asleep. He wanted to know whether I thought that that was acceptable. Rather shocked, I asked him whether he had used the 100% solution directly from the bottle. That is exactly ıe had done. I then asked whether the son had responded to the concentration with severe skin irritation but the answer was no. had tolerated it well and the pain and the inflammation had abated .ickly. This shows that the effects vary widely from one individual to ɩnother and that DMSO is a very 'forgiving' substance.

Case: A.G., 6 years old, suffered from a chronic inflammation of the ear canal and eczema on the auricle. His parents said that he was often unable to sleep because of this. The boy was able to sleep after just a single application of a few drops of a 50% DMSO solution and the whole problem disappeared within a few days.

Case: D.S., 3 years old, had had a bad cold, a cough and a fever for a number of days. Then his condition suddenly changed, with the previous symptoms disappearing only to be replaced by a severe earache. This kind of 'wandering' is common and inflammations of the middle ear are regarded as a complication resulting from more trivial infections. The child's mother sought my advice and little D. was given a few drops of a 35% DMSO solution in the bad ear. Her tears of pain dried up within a few minutes and she smiled broadly. Of course, the little darling then started to complain vigorously about the itching, but that was a sign of revived spirits.

Elevated intracranial pressure See Spinal cord injuries

Embolism See Infarctions

Epilepsy See Developmental disorders in children

Eye diseases (see also Age-related macular degeneration)
Eye specialists have used and continue to use DMSO by itself and in combination with other substances to treat a range of eye diseases with great success. These conditions include macular degeneration, macular oedema, uveitis due to trauma (inflammation of the middle structures of the eye), cataract, glaucoma, and various retina diseases. Cataracts can be treated very simply by applying a drop of DMSO solution (use sterile isotonic water) directly into the eye. Other eye treatments should be left to eye specialists. Excellent results have been achieved by locally administering a special mixture of DMSO and superoxide dismutase

(SOD) to treat glaucoma. The function of the SOD enzyme, a biocatalyst that is also naturally present in all aerobic organisms, is explained in Chapter 2.5.1.

Furthermore, it has often been observed that patients who take DMSO to treat musculoskeletal pains also report noticeable improvements in any eye conditions they may have suffered from. A patient suffering from advanced retinal degeneration (retinitis pigmentosa) reported a spectacular recovery in his eyesight while undergoing DMSO treatment for other reasons. As a result, a clinical study was started at the University of Oregon to research this phenomenon. A further 50 patients with retina diseases were treated by Dr Robert Hill in the early 1970s and the overall results were very encouraging. The patients' visual acuity, field of vision and night vision improved or stabilised. I recently treated a female patient suffering from muscle pains in the neck using a DMSO solution and she reported a few days later with great surprise that on the following morning she could suddenly see clearly even without her old glasses. In this case, DMSO's muscle-relaxing effect presumably played a part alongside its regenerative properties.

When treating the eyes directly using a drop solution, make certain that the ingredients are as sterile as possible and ensure that the solution is strongly diluted. Formula suggestions for such applications are given in Chapter 2; you will need 5 grams of purified DMSO mixed into a 1000ml isotonic saline infusion. The quantity you require for the eye drops can be extracted from that using a sterile syringe / cannula.

Foot problems

Morton Walker,[19] himself a podiatrist, has compiled a long list of foot problems that can be treated using DMSO, either by itself or in combination with other medications. He calls this 'foot care medicine'. The list includes bunions, hammertoe, corns, calluses, warts, ingrowing toenails, fungal nail, athlete's foot (see Athlete's foot), foot odour, ballerina-foot pattern, metatarsalgia (painful metatarsal bones), flat foot, calcaneal spur (see Calcaneal spur) and sprained ankles. Some of these complaints, when they become chronic, may need surgical treatment. However, acute pains, inflammations, hardening, swelling etc. can all be alleviated using DMSO. Apply it liberally to the affected area. Fungal nail can be treated usinsg a combination of DMSO and MMS (see Athlete's foot). When combined with DMSO, MMS penetrates the tissue more deeply thereby improving its efficacy.

Fractured bones See Sports injuries

Gout

Acute attacks of gout are caused by elevated uric acid levels in the blood. Standard values are about 3 to 6mg/dL for women and 4 to 7mg/dL for men. It is only in hominids (humans, apes) that uric acid is found in the blood in such quantities; the values are up to ten times higher in hominids than in all other mammals. Uric acid is eliminated mainly through the kidneys, although some is also eliminated via the skin and bowels. Since uric acid has been shown to elevate blood pressure, it has been speculated that the partial retention of this substance (up to the standard values) might have made it possible for the more developed mammals (i.e. humans, chimpanzees, gorillas and orangutans) to walk upright. After all, it is vital to ensure a sufficient supply of blood to the brain – in defiance of gravity – for that to happen.

Uric acid levels in the blood exceeding 7mg/dL can, in combination with other factors (cold, liquid deficiency, nicotine, alcohol, etc.), cause the substance to crystalize from the solution (the blood) in which it is transported, and be deposited in parts of the body that have a poor blood supply. You might remember this principle from 'crystal cultivation' experiments in your school days. This occurs primarily in the toes, especially in the base joint of the right big toe, leading to the typical symptoms of a gout attack, including severe pain, redness and swelling. In short, the uric acid crystals – as a foreign body – trigger an intense inflammatory reaction.

Treatment using DMSO: DMSO's anti-inflammatory, pain-relieving and regenerative capacities quickly bring relief to the gouty toe. A 75 to 80% solution is brushed or sprayed onto the affected area. Repeat as often as necessary. In addition to this immediate measure you should not forget that gout is, essentially, a metabolic disorder. Nutrition, circulation and exercise habits must be assessed, and changes must be made to lower levels of uric acid so as to avoid further gout attacks in the long-term.

Gum inflammations See Aphthae

Haematoma See Sports injuries

Headaches / migraines See Pains

Herpes / herpes zoster See Shingles

Hyperactivity / hyperkinesia See Developmental disorders in children

Hypertension / high blood pressure See Arteriosclerosis

Infarctions

Infarctions always require immediate treatment because of the risk that the tissue damage could advance and become permanent. They are caused by local deficiencies in the supply of oxygen due to circulation problems. Blood clots (embolisms), deposits (plaque, uric acid crystals, etc.) and injuries are all possible causes. The most important intensive care measures, therefore, are oxygen administration, improving the rheological property of the blood (blood flow rate) and / or removal of the congestive thrombus through surgery or medication (thrombectomy, thrombolysis). Life-threating infarctions include heart attacks, strokes, renal infarction, mesenteric infarction (abdominal organs), lung infarction (usually lung embolism) and hepatic infarction. There have been a number of cases in which tissue damaged as a result of an oxygen deficiency has improved significantly after DMSO treatment. In cases of stroke, DMSO has helped patients to regain cognitive skills such as walking and talking much more quickly. This is not surprising considering what we know regarding DMSO's oxygen diffusion property and its general capacity to transport substances into and out of cells. This also has a positive effect on the repair and regeneration of the area affected by the infarction. Even though it is widely known that the best results are achieved when DMSO is administered as soon as possible following a stroke, as far as I know the 'stroke units' that have recently been established in order to give specialised treatment for stroke patients do not use DMSO infusions.

Morton Walker[19] lists a range of causes for cerebral infarctions. The most common are acute strokes, which are, in turn, triggered by arteriosclerosis, high blood pressure or a combination of both. Other potential causes include: embolisms caused by fat deposits, entrapped air (the much-feared decompression effect when diving) and fragments of blood clots that can be formed by damage to heart ventricles (left). This kind of damage to the ventricle, in turn, can be the result of sclerosis plaque, heart valve deposits, bacterial endocarditis, rheumatic diseases of the endocardium, and heart attacks, or they can occur following heart operations. DMSO can, in all these cases, stop the damaging chain reaction that is set off by reduced tissue perfusion and that ultimately leads to the destruction of the affected nerve cells. DMSO reduces platelet aggregation, thereby preventing the formation of further thrombi. DMSO promotes the release of the specific prostaglandin (a tissue hormone) that expands the neighbouring blood vessels, thereby addressing and reversing the oxygen deficiency. DMSO also has a vasodilating effect of its own. Through its cell-protecting and regenerative effects, DMSO supports energy production in the area affected by the deficient supply. As a result, the cells have sufficient time to reach a stable condition and avert any further damage. It has been proven in countless clinical studies on animals and humans that DMSO treatment for infarctions should be given as quickly as possible and at suitably high doses if a cure is to be brought about.

DMSO infusions are recommended in all acute cases of vascular occlusion. Up to 1 gram of DMSO per kilogram of body weight can be administered as an aqueous solution in an isotonic electrolyte infusion solution as soon as possible after the onset of the disease. This should only be carried out by experienced health professionals. A suitable quantity of infusion solution must be used to ensure that the concentrations of DMSO do not become too high. Depending on body weight and on the illness, you can use 500ml or 1000ml infusions. In cases of serious illnesses such as infarctions we do not administer gradually increasing doses of DMSO; the high total quantity is administered from the outset. The dose can then be decreased at the first signs of improvement.

Infections

The word 'infection' is defined in the *Brockhaus*, an authoritative German encyclopaedia, as follows: 'Infection, contagion: an invasion of pathogens (bacteria, viruses, fungi, parasites) in the body'.

That means, firstly, that infections 'only' involve the establishment of microorganisms in the (physical) body. Officially that is still not a disease because this process does not necessarily lead to noticeable or measurable symptoms. When such silent, symptom-free infection processes lead to temporary or lifelong immunity, we speak of occult immunisation.

In contrast, a (real) infectious disease, and the reactions and responses of our immune system to foreign invaders, is characterised by general symptoms such as fever, night sweats, reduced energy, increased secretion and signs of inflammation. Today we know that neither the symptomatic nor the silent infections are always dealt with successfully. Chronic processes that result from the incomplete destruction of the invading microorganism can develop. Developments may be noticeable or can proceed clandestinely, for example when the 'enemy' has been able to hide or when it evolves through different stages of development, or when our immune systems are weakened by medications or other illnesses. It is also possible for all the viruses or bacteria to be killed but that the body fails to eliminate the particles of enemy detritus glued to the body's own immune structures (antigen antibody complexes). All these incomplete immune reactions are, to put it simply, thought to be responsible for a large number of chronic secondary diseases, including severe conditions and 'incurable' diseases (according to mainstream medicine). These include allergies, autoimmune disorders, recurring infections, and cancer. That is why the following two points are important for us and for our pets.

Firstly, we should always make sure that the immune system, our immune cells, are in good order. It is particularly important that the intestinal flora is healthy and this can only be achieved in the long term by eating a good, natural diet. Countless millennia of evolution, over the course of which humans and other mammals have constantly developed, cannot be distorted and changed by a few years of industrial food processing – I hope that that is clear! We are only considering a period of sixty years during which it has become normal to fill our fridges and cupboards with machine-produced convenience foods that have chemicals added to them.

What do you think? 'It could be as long as eighty years.' That is inconsequential. Even if it had been a hundred years or two hundred years, that is not even the blink of an eye in terms of the speed with which genetic shifts occur within a single species. The human body, and especially the digestive system and the glands that belong to it, does not have the means at its disposal to detoxify industrially produced foods or to use that food to nourish and heal itself. Read more on this topic in 'Guidelines for healthy living' in Dr Antje Oswald's *The MMS Handbook: Your Health in Your Hands*. She once wrote to me saying that there are unfortunate fellow human beings who do not even know that lettuces do not grow in plastic bags or do not know what a carrot looks like ...

Secondly, in cases of an infection (or infectious disease), the function of the immune system must be supported. To support means to imitate its natural functions and to relieve the burden on the system. The burden can best be relieved by using common measures such as increasing the liquid intake (e.g. detoxifying teas), plenty of rest, and an improved diet. Immune cell functions can be imitated by taking oxidative substances, as was explained in detail in the section entitled 'DMSO and MMS'. In this context – and I do not mind repeating this point because it is so important – it is irrelevant whether the problem is caused by invading microorganisms or by enemies from within such as (mutated) cancer cells. Antibiotics, cytostatics, chemotherapy medicine – none of these can provide this kind of imitation. To make matter worse, they all damage the body's own cells and the intestinal flora to varying degrees, thereby leading to a weakening of the immune system in the long term.

Taking DMSO, which has an anti-inflammatory and immune-modulating effect, not only inhibits the growth of bacteria, viruses and fungi, but it also plays a vital role in assisting oxidative substances that are administered alongside it (MMS or hydrogen peroxide) to penetrate the tissue more effectively. DMSO can be used to naturally support and shorten the period of regeneration and repair necessary after an infection has been fought off. To do so, follow the instructions in Chapter 2 regarding staggered administration of MMS. Alternatively the substances can be administered via the skin or by infusion. Starting with a basic dose (0.05g per kilogram of body weight), increase the quantity of DMSO administered daily according to your needs.

Infections of the middle ear See Ear infections

Inflammation of the throat See Respiratory tract infections

Insect bites

Wasp, bee and mosquito stings are unpleasant, painful and itchy at the best of times. To make matters worse, many people have an allergic disposition and have inflammatory overreactions to such incidents. The injury to the skin caused by such bites can also lead to (secondary) bacterial infections. Allergic reactions are discussed in a separate section. Other symptoms of insect bites can also be treated effectively using

DMSO. The most suitable application method is to spray an appropriate dilution of DMSO solution. DMSO concentration in these preparations is determined by which part of the body is affected. When treating the head and face start by using low concentrations (30 to 50%), use medium concentrations (50 to 65%) when treating the torso, and use higher concentrations (60 to 80%) when treating below the waistline.

What can DMSO do in such cases? The anti-inflammatory and pain-relieving effects quickly cause the itching, swelling and pain to abate. The sooner the DMSO solution is applied after the bite, the less marked and developed the typical symptoms become. In addition, any insect poisons that might have entered the body are broken down far more quickly with the aid of DMSO. This effect can be understood in at least two different ways. Firstly, we are familiar with the 'carrier effect', which causes toxin molecules to be 'enveloped', making it easier for them to cross through biomembranes such as cell and vessel walls. Secondly, the influx of bipolar, antioxidant DMSO instantly brings about a dilution in the local concentration of toxic substances, whose power to cause damage is thereby neutralised. Combining DMSO with oxidative substances such as MMS / CDS and hydrogen peroxide is also a good option as that can heal insect bites even more quickly. If you decide on this option, first spray the MMS or H_2O_2 solution, then administer the DMSO in a suitable dilution (see Chapter 2.5.1).

Irritable bowel syndrome

This condition is a diagnosis of exclusion. That means, first of all, that tests should be carried out to see whether other (more serious) reasons for the typical symptoms (e.g. abdominal pain, fatigue, malaise) can be found. Ultimately, a diagnosis of irritable bowel syndrome means that imaging and other diagnostic measures have not been able to detect any signs of disease. The good news, then, is that these complaints are not an early stage of other severe gastrointestinal diseases. The bad news is that no one really knows what causes it and how it should be treated. Symptoms vary greatly from one individual to another. Some patients suffer from diarrhoea while others become constipated. There are often overlaps with partly psychogenic conditions such as fibromyalgia, and with food intolerances, allergies, damaged intestinal flora, and hormone disturbances (see the section on Premenstrual syndrome (PMS)). Because the onset of the symptoms is usually characterised by a sudden change in bowel habits, diseases such as Crohn's disease, ulcerative colitis, intestinal polyps and carcinomas must be excluded. Depending on the specific symptoms, mainstream treatments include laxatives, antidepressants and muscle relaxants (Buscopan®) with or without painkillers (e.g. paracetamol, metamizole).

Because of its spectrum of pharmacological effects, DMSO is suitable as a treatment for irritable bowel syndrome and the complaints associated with it. The most important of these effects are pain relief, muscle relaxation and detoxification support. The administration of DMSO as a treatment for this set of symptoms has shown clearly that it has holistic balancing and gently modulating effects. Some patients report that they feel something is 'missing' when they stop taking DMSO, even if they cannot describe exactly all the beneficial effects they had observed while they were taking it. Other common natural medications for bowel regulation can and should be used to cleanse the intestines and to support the intestinal flora. These include psyllium husks, inulin and right-turning lactic acid. I have also had good results using meditative exercises to stretch the musculature of the torso. In accordance with the patient's constitution (iris diagnosis), homeopathic and complex-homeopathic remedies can be used to treat the cause or as a supportive measure. DMSO can be taken via the skin, in a drink or by infusion. If the patient is suffering from serious bowel or digestive problems, it might be better not to start the treatment using a drink solution. Depending on the development of the symptoms, the initial dose is 0.05g per kg of body weight, increasing gradually.

ITP / Werlhof's disease

Idiopathic thrombocytopenic purpura (also known as immune thrombocytopenia), a low blood platelet count due to an autoimmune reaction, can occur in acute form (mostly in children) and in chronic form (> 6 months, mostly in adults). It is often noted that this large-scale destruction of thrombocytes is preceded by a viral (e.g. glandular fever, cytomegalovirus, fifth disease) or a bacterial (*Helicobacter pylori* stomach bacteria) infection. A temporal connection between (viral) infections and the later appearance of autoimmune reactions is often observed in these diseases of 'self-destruction' and they are regarded as complications during the healing phase of the infection. ITP can lead to thrombocyte values of below 15,000 platelets per μL (microliter) of blood. A normal value is between 150,000 and 450,000 per μL. This condition hugely diminishes blood coagulation with consequences such as spontaneous bleeding in the skin (petechiae), in the mucous membranes (nose, gum, gastrointestinal bleeding), in the joints, and in other organs such as the kidneys and brain. The mainstream medical treatments for this condition are high doses of cortisone, immunoglobulin treatment (sometimes combined with the administration of antibodies) and as a last resort, the removal of the spleen.

From a holistic perspective, we are dealing primarily with a dysfunction of the immune system. In alternative medicine, one treatment option for such a problem is to establish or support a healthy intestinal flora, which plays a fundamentally important role in 'training' immune defence cells throughout the body. Any other treatments that modulate the immune system can also be considered. It would be particularly suitable to administer DMSO, perhaps at first in combination with the detoxifying and pathogen-killing substance MMS, preferably orally or as an infusion. Because ITP can be a protracted illness, patients must show a certain level of staying power, particularly when it comes to administering long-term DMSO treatments.

Case: Mr J. M., 38 years old, developed chronic ITP in the spring of 2011. As is so often the case, the huge decrease in his thrombocyte counts went undetected for a long time. After all, you do not usually go for a blood test every two weeks. At times the thrombocyte count fell below 20,000 per µL. The initial treatment involving high doses of cortisone brought about a temporary stabilisation at around 70,000 per µL. Then the number of thrombocytes began to drop again in stages. Since the doctors had threatened to remove the patient's spleen, he sought alternative advice on how the illness could be treated. I recommended he take DMSO. This led to a swift improvement and the blood count increased to 87,000 per µL within a week. Since we were dealing with an immune response, I also suggested he take MMS in parallel with the DMSO, 2 to 3 times a day at increasing doses starting with 2 drops. He continued conscientiously with this over many weeks, reaching a dose of 3 x 6 drops. However, he stopped taking DMSO after two weeks because the odour became a problem. There followed a period of considerable fluctuation in the blood values, which were taken every 1 to 2 weeks by his doctor. In the end I supported him in the decision to undergo the antibody treatment that had been suggested because I felt that that would give him some reassurance. However, the patient himself insisted on continuing to take MMS without interruption. He was, at this stage, still not ready to restart taking DMSO. The case is still ongoing and as we go to press the latest figures we have show that the blood count has risen to 184,000 per µL. Even though the success in this case cannot be wholly attributed to DMSO, we see very clearly that it is worth exhausting all the alternative treatment options when it comes to protracted, chronic diseases.

Joint inflammation

Joint inflammation can be caused by a number of different circumstances. It can develop as a complication after surgical or therapeutic (joint injections) intervention, or can be caused by overstraining, rheumatism, or accumulation of deposits. Inflamed joints is one of the main fields of applications for DMSO. Its unique ability to penetrate biological membranes is of particular importance in this context. There are no blood vessels inside the joint capsules. As a result, the processes of supplying nutrients and eliminating waste such as metabolic by-products and inflammatory toxins are far less effective than in other parts of the body. Repair processes are difficult and are undertaken by means of diffusion processes, which are very slow. These repair processes are highly sensitive to temperature, substance concentrations and irritation caused by repetitive movements. When joint pain causes the patient to try to protect the joint by adopting relieving postures, the vicious circle is complete because this stagnation limits the diffusion process. DMSO really comes to the fore in such cases, playing all its trump cards. Its numerous pharmacological properties, which were listed in Chapter 1.2.3, play an important part in healing joint inflammation because it can penetrate with ease through skin, musculature and the joint capsule to reach the location of the inflammation.

In his book[19] Morton Walker describes the case of a patient who suffered from rheumatoid bone inflammation in both knees and who could only arrive at his doctor's surgery with the aid of two crutches. Lucas Sheinholtz, then 52 years old, had been suffering from this debilitating arthritis for more than ten years. A number of attempts to treat the condition using cortisone injections had brought no relief. A professor working at the hospital where Sheinholtz was being treated had taken delivery of a batch of DMSO and had decided to use it to try to help patients who had not seen any results from other treatments. He advised Sheinholtz's doctor to brush the substance onto his patient's knees. The doctor had no experience of working with DMSO and repeatedly applied DMSO as soon as the previous dose had been absorbed. After 15 to 20 minutes the patient no longer felt any pain and he could walk without his crutches. When he returned a week later he reported that the left knee had remained completely free of pain. The right knee, which had been badly swollen and hyperthermic the previous week, was still slightly painful. The doctor repeated the DMSO application and has not seen that patient since.

Learning difficulties See Developmental disorders in children

Liver diseases

Liver inflammation (hepatitis), fatty liver, liver cirrhosis and congested liver are all included under this broad umbrella term. Under these conditions the liver, as the multifunctioning super-organ that it is, is unable to perform its metabolic tasks properly, resulting in the destruction of liver cells. Dysfunction of this kind can be detected in laboratory tests showing elevated 'liver values'. These are specific enzymes that are used as a criterion for evaluating the condition of the liver. Acute viral inflammations are, by law, notifiable illnesses. However, hepatitis can also be caused by an autoimmune problem. The most common causes of fatty liver are long-term alcohol misuse and overeating. Both can lead to irreversible liver cirrhosis, as can congested liver, which is usually originally caused by cardiac insufficiency. Even though the liver tissue has an amazing capacity for regeneration, it is important to eliminate causative factors (e.g. alcohol) at an early stage and / or to treat the underlying illness.

DMSO, as a regenerative substance, can certainly take an important place as a basic medication in this context. For liver diseases I recommend either taking DMSO via the skin or as an infusion because by taking it in this way DMSO does not pass through the portal venous system. DMSO, when taken as a drink solution, can temporarily increase the stress placed on the liver. Start treatment using doses of 0.1 gram of DMSO per kilogram of body weight, increasing gradually according to the patient's condition.

Macular degeneration See Age-related macular degeneration (AMD)

Mental disabilities See Developmental disorders in children

Migraines See Pains

Multiple sclerosis (see also Chronic fatigue syndrome)

Multiple sclerosis (MS), in contrast to other common diseases that affect the central nervous system (dementia, Parkinson's, etc.), involves inflammation of the neurons. That is the origin of the name 'encephalo-myelitis disseminata', which indicates that the condition involves a number of centres of inflammation scattered throughout the brain and spinal cord. These processes lead, usually in episodic bursts, to damage to the insulating covers of the nerve cell axons (white matter), thereby losing their ability to conduct electrical impulses to a greater or lesser degree. The symptoms vary from individual to individual, ranging from minor dysfunction to a complete inability to walk or move. It is still not clear what exactly causes MS despite the vast amount of research that has been done on the condition. The inflammation is, however, clearly triggered by an immune response, with the body's own immune cells attacking the covers of the cell axons. The current scientific data points towards a possible link to viral or bacterial diseases suffered during childhood. The main suspect is the Epstein–Barr virus (glandular fever), although the initial infection suffered in the past may have run its course without the patient noticing any of the typical symptoms. That, of course, makes it all the more difficult to establish a link. It is assumed that such infections can lead to a dysfunction of the immune cells, to state it in very general terms. Today, it is increasingly thought that other diseases are also caused in a similar way. There are other, very different hypotheses on how and why MS develops, including reactions to vaccinations, vitamin D levels and excess loads of environmental toxins and stimulants. When viewed holistically, the stories patients tell often reveal a strong connection between the disease and psychological stress. This is not surprising considering the many other immune system diseases that involve a psychological element.

We have already learned that DMSO has an anti-inflammatory effect and regulates the immune system. Drawing from the positive experiences that MS patients have had with DMSO in the past, DMSO's holistic and regenerative effect is very clearly seen; it heals in a natural and powerful way. Appropriate quantities of DMSO should be taken by applying it to large areas of the skin, drinking a diluted solution, or taken via an infusion.

Russian doctors published the results of DMSO use in the treatment of 34 MS patients in 1984.[68] The authors came to the conclusion that DMSO is a good treatment for MS because it has a positive effect on the immune system, has an anti-allergenic effect and repairs damaged tissue. The treatment proved to be particularly effective for patients with relapsing MS. Progress was inconsistent for patients suffering from the rapidly progressive form of MS. No side effects were observed. The healing effect of DMSO was attributed to the processes of remineralisation (reforming the myelin sheaths of the nerve fibres), the reduction of oedemas, and improvements in neuro-dynamic impulse transmission.

Muscle pains See Pains

Muscle weakness / muscular dystrophies in children
See Developmental disorders in children

Myasthenia gravis   (see also Neurodegenerative diseases)

This is an autoimmune disease in which the nerve cell receptors are blocked and destroyed. This hinders the transmission of electrical impulses or signals between the nerve cells and the (skeletal) musculature. The muscles become fatigued very quickly and require long periods of rest to recover. That is the meaning of the disease's Latin name 'myasthenia gravis', which can be translated as severe muscle weakness. Since this muscle weakness is caused by strain, the symptoms typically worsen significantly over the course of a day. If the condition develops it can lead to outright paralysis that, in the worst cases, can affect breathing and swallowing. In the initial phases, it is usually the eyelid muscles, the expressive muscles and the oral muscles that are affected. It is still not known what causes this condition. Women between the ages of 20 and 40 are most likely to be affected. In some cases a connection can be established between the onset of the disease and previous infections or thymus conditions. In the latter case, treatment initially involves the surgical removal of the thymus, after which many patients recover. Otherwise, cortisone and other substances that suppress the immune system are used, as in other autoimmune disorders, to try to eliminate the immune system dysfunction. Other standard treatments for myasthenia gravis include the removal of the autoantibodies by exchanging the blood plasma and immunoglobulin administration. A targeted drug treatment can be administered by giving synthetic enzyme inhibitors (cholinesterase inhibitors). This increases the locally available quantity of the neurotransmitter that is responsible for transmitting the neural command signals to the muscles (acetylcholine). However, these medications have a number of undesirable effects including gastrointestinal cramp, vomiting, increased salivation, low heart rate, narrowing of the bronchi, and eye muscle dysfunction. They should not be taken during pregnancy or when breastfeeding.

As explained in the sections on other autoimmune disorders, we can assume that there is a holistic or multifactorial origin to this kind of malfunction or overreaction by the immune cells. This is already clear from the fact that symptoms are compounded by negative environmental influences, stress / worry and infections. If the road to this illness has taken a certain period of time, the road out of this illness may well take just as long. As part of that journey detoxification, and ridding yourself of burdens of all kinds, should help you towards finding a new balance and true healing. This is also true for the balance of normal immune processes. DMSO, as we learned in the previous chapter, can be an important basic remedy in this regard. It has an immune modulation effect and it supports detoxification processes. It supports cell membranes (and nerve and muscle cells) and it inhibits the destruction of neurotransmitters. And all this from a medicine that is easy to tolerate.

DMSO is taken both internally and externally in the treatment of myasthenia gravis. DMSO (60 to 75% aqueous solution) can be brushed onto individual limbs or muscle groups affected by the condition. At the same time, DMSO can be taken internally as a drink solution or as an infusion, starting with about 3.5 grams a day. Depending on the progress made, the dose is then adjusted for the individual and supported by other appropriate measures. If cortisone is used, bear in mind that DMSO will significantly increase its effect.

Nail inflammations

Nail inflammations are usually very painful and often lead to purulent discharge. They can be caused by ingrowing nails, injuries caused by nail implements, and from wearing shoes that are too small. When applied locally, DMSO solutions quickly alleviate the swelling and pain. The inflammation disappears after a number of applications of a 75% preparation (often by the second day); it can be applied in drops onto the nail bed using a cotton wool pad. You should take care when using nail scissors to avoid causing further injuries.

Nervousness in children See Developmental disorders in children

Neuralgia

Neuralgia is another term for nerve pains. They are caused by irritation or damage to the peripheral nerves or nerve axons. The peripheral nervous system consists of all the areas not included in the central nervous system (which includes the brain and spinal cord). Peripheral nerves, i.e. nerves that directly connect to organs, muscles and skin, can easily be strained by mechanical pressure (e.g. carpal tunnel syndrome) because they are not protected by bone. Infections (shingles), inflammations (neuritis), supply disruptions (polyneuropathy) or radiation can lead to damage and resulting pain in the nerves of the outer parts of the body. Neuralgias often develop as a complication during or after the healing phase of other underlying conditions. A typical example of this is trigeminal neuralgia (tic douloureux), which can develop after an inflammation of the middle ear, causing painful spasms in the muscles of the face. Neuralgias can be temporary or can become chronic and can cause immense suffering for many patients. The triggers and the duration of the painful attacks vary considerably, resulting in patients feeling a tormenting sense of insecurity and sometimes causing them to take absurd measures in the hope of avoiding the symptoms.

If possible, the underlying illness is treated either curatively or on the level of the symptoms. Mainstream medicine uses a scale to measure and treat pain, employing increasingly powerful painkillers. Depending on the advancement or the responsiveness of the pain syndrome, medicines from the opium family, or medicines also used to treat depression and epilepsy, are employed. If these measures fail to control the problem the patient sometimes has to undergo an operation ... if they agree to it. Many choose to do so because they see no other way out of their suffering. Some patients even commit suicide because of this condition.

You will already have read in the introduction that DMSO was used by many thousands of Americans in the 1960s mainly to treat pain. This was the main field of application in which the pharmaceutical industry was interested in getting DMSO officially approved for commercial sale. DMSO is an excellent painkiller: it works quickly and can be used locally by anyone. Since neuralgias usually develop close to the surface, external application in the form of an aqueous solution is the method of choice. The affected area (for example one half of the face, the ribs, or the wrist) is brushed or sprayed liberally. Take care to prevent the liquid from getting into the eyes. As explained in Chapter 2, lower concentrations of DMSO solution are used above the waistline compared with the amount used for treatments below the waistline. You should always begin with concentrations below 60% when treating the face, just to be on the safe side. You can work with concentrations of 75% or higher when working on the wrists or the legs (e.g. peroneal nerve irritation). In addition to the swift pain relief that DMSO brings about by inhibiting the transmission of signals to certain nerve cell fibres, the anti-inflammatory and regenerative effects can also be significant. Neuralgias are feared more than anything because of the startling and unpredictable way they occur. They can be triggered by sensitivity to other factors such as sudden changes in temperature or touch. This often leads to patients isolating themselves, hardly leaving their homes. Such a retreat from society intensifies their suffering even further. However, these chronically fickle symptoms probably result from inflammation or a long-term deficiency in the supply to the tissue. These triggers are quickly healed by DMSO treatment. That is why treatment should not be discontinued once the pains abate after the first application. It is worth persisting with the treatment so that the nerve damage can be repaired as completely as possible.

Neurodegenerative diseases

This category of diseases includes Parkinson's, Alzheimer's / dementia, amyotrophic lateral sclerosis, Creutzfeldt–Jakob disease and other similar conditions, Huntington's chorea, spinal muscular atrophy and many others. As the name indicates, these diseases are all characterised by a loss of nerve cells. Depending on the actual function of the respective nerve cells or the affected area of the brain, the disease causes progressively more severe limitations to brain function, movement or perception. 'Stand-in' substances such as Alzheimer's plaque can also become embedded where the decayed tissue was previously. The resulting, observable symptoms of neurodegeneration therefore vary a great deal from patient to patient. The causes and the development of cell degradation vary greatly and are still not entirely understood. However, there is a statistical link between neurodegenerative diseases and 'diseases of civilisation' such as high blood pressure, adult-onset diabetes and elevated blood fat values. Or to put it another way, it has often been observed that a healthy, natural lifestyle generally reduces your risk of having such illnesses. Ensuring an adequate supply of vitamin B, oxygen and antioxidant phytochemicals has a significant protective effect against the disease. That supports the theory that the disease begins with local metabolic dysfunctions in the nerve tissue. These lead to diffusion and supply problems, causing the cell and matrix milieu to become acidic and oxidative.

These are all key words that should remind us of DMSO. Mainstream medicines – i.e. medicines produced by the pharmaceutical industry to treat some of these diseases – are rather ineffective. 'Promising candidates' for the treatment of Alzheimer's have been in the pipeline for many years but when put to the test they have failed to convince. The same is true for Parkinson's disease. The only useful measures are usually movement therapy and providing support for the patient's family. That can alleviate symptoms and sometimes slow down the progress of the disease.

We know from the successes we have experienced when treating polyneuropathy (my own father among them) that DMSO has a regenerative effect on the nerve cells and their functions. Neurons that have already been destroyed cannot, of course, be brought back to life. However, healthy cells and axons that are still functioning can adjust, as we know from neuroscientific research, to the increased demands made on them, compensating for the loss in numbers to some extent. It is, therefore, worth fighting for each and every cell, and to choose a holistic approach. DMSO is an excellent antioxidant and it protects cells. It improves the supply of nutrients to the cells through vasodilation, membrane activity and better diffusion. Oxygen concentrations are raised and the cell functions are stabilised. Acetylcholine, a neurotransmitter that is extremely important for the brain, can become deficient as a result of tissue degradation. DMSO can elevate acetylcholine levels because it inhibits the enzymes that break down the neurotransmitter. DMSO can be administered internally or externally depending on the stage and development of the disease. You will find guidelines on appropriate doses and concentrations in Chapter 2. Skin applications, drink solutions and infusions can be combined as you see fit. Other measures should be tried and taken alongside DMSO. There is positive data available on ginkgo biloba extracts, compounds from green and black tea as well as other plant antioxidants. Galactose appears to be a promising treatment. This is a biochemical sister-substance to glucose, which is very important for cells in the central nervous system. Galactose and glucose are components of lactose which is present in breast milk and is partly responsible for the quick development of the brain in infants. Because this sugar, unlike glucose, is not dependent on insulin to reach the energy centres of the cells, I also like to use it as part of a holistic treatment for adult-onset diabetes. It has astoundingly positive effects when integrated into a treatment programme. Unfortunately, galactose is expensive (about £65 to £110 pounds per 500g) and as far as I know is not available as an infusion solution. This is an important point because when absorbed through the intestine, a certain percentage is immediately converted into glucose so we have to employ certain tricks as we administer the substance. Galactose, when used as part of a treatment for neurodegenerative diseases, is a good way of supplying energy to cells that are stressed and 'hungry' due to metabolic dysfunctions. That enables the cell to carry out its own detoxification and regeneration processes. The standard dosage recommendation for oral intake is up to 6 grams twice a day (a teaspoon is approximately 3 grams).

Other treatment options include dietary changes, exercise and, most importantly, mental activity. Unfortunately, the scientific discovery that television and crossword puzzles have a negative effect on the course of the disease has still not been widely reported. Because patients retreat from society permanently, these two 'consumption-oriented' hobbies are often all that remain for them. However, if patients want to remain mentally fit for as long as possible they need to undertake other, very different activities. Firstly, scientifically approved 'brain-exercise' books and DVDs are now available. Secondly, occupying themselves with appropriate educational topics and, most importantly, having stimulating conversations with various people have been proven to have a beneficial effect on the condition.

Operations

Surgical operations place an exceptional strain on our bodies. In addition to the healing work the body has to carry out on all levels afterwards, the main problem is the formation of external and internal scars. It is therefore wise to question the necessity of any planned operation. If no other alternative is available, prepare the body for surgery using DMSO. This can be done by administering DMSO locally onto areas that are to be operated on, by drinking DMSO solutions or by infusion. Procaine / alkaline infusions (see Chapter 2.5.2) are also a good way to prepare for surgery – on the spine, for example – and to support recovery. This helps regeneration processes, alleviates scar formation and reduces the risk of adhesions. Because of its anticoagulant effect, DMSO should not be used on the day of the operation.

It is worth asking whether the surgeon could wear powder-free surgical gloves because these particles can cause long-term scar disturbances if they enter the wound. When administered as soon as possible after the operation, DMSO supports the healing process noticeably and helps to ease pain. It is important to treat the external scar as soon as possible so that no disturbance field forms. One excellent method is to flood the skin surface with an alkaline procaine solution after having liberally moistened the scar area with a 60 to 70% DMSO solution beforehand. The mixture containing 1 to 2% procaine in a sodium bicarbonate solution is injected into the skin along the stitch using a very fine needle (size 18 or 20) so that the wheals that form flow into each other.

Incidentally, this method can be used to treat all scars, no matter how old they are. Almost without exception, patients report very positive responses to this remedial measure – such as getting rejuvenating sleep once more, or feeling a new sense of inner balance – either immediately or within a few days. What is just as important in my view, however, is the healing of chronic irritation and pain in the scarred area and the joy patients feel regarding cosmetic improvements. The appearance of old scars can be improved considerably using a number of other additional measures, all of which are easy to administer. In some cases the scars become almost invisible.

Osteitis

Osteitis, or inflammation of the bone, can affect any part of the bone, including the bone marrow, the bone tissue itself or the periosteum. The condition is caused by infections – most often bacterial but sometimes viral or fungal – following injuries and operations. Mainstream medical doctors often prefer prompt surgical intervention because there is no guarantee that antibiotics will reach the site of the infection. Unfortunately these operations are often not as effective as would be desired even though they are constantly being developed. As a result, it is almost inevitable that the disease becomes protracted. A (combination) treatment using DMSO is a good alternative. You can administer it in combination with mainstream antimicrobial medicines and / or cortisone, or you can administer it in combination with a tried-and-tested oxidant such as MMS. The latter approach is also recommended in painful cases of aseptic bone inflammations (i.e. not caused by microorganisms). DMSO can find its way into all areas of tissues, exerting its anti-inflammatory effect as it does so. It also carries the other medicines with it wherever it goes. Patients benefit from DMSO's pain-relieving effects, from improved mobility, and from the reduced need for relieving postures.

DMSO is taken internally or applied externally, depending on which part of the body is affected. Of course, you can take external and internal (drink / infusion) administrations simultaneously. Since many bones are very close to the surface you can often opt for a topical administration. Brush or spray DMSO solution onto a large area of skin. Higher concentrations of DMSO can be used on the extremities (arms and legs) than on the torso or the head and face. If you decide to use DMSO in combination with a suitable antibiotic, the antibiotic (dissolved in DMSO) can also be applied to the skin. If the antibiotic is intended for oral administration, its efficacy / tissue penetration is improved when DMSO is taken internally at the same time. The same is also true of alternative bactericides such as MMS. When taking DMSO and MMS, the two substances should be taken separately, one soon after the other.

Osteomyelitis See Osteitis

Pain

Headache, toothache, muscle pain, joint and back pain, pain following operations and injuries, menstrual cramp ... the list could continue. Sales of over-the-counter and prescription painkillers are huge and, despite criticisms of this trend from various quarters over many years, advertising campaigns are still undertaken to encourage growth in this market. Media images everywhere show that taking synthetic, chemical painkillers will make you happy and successful. For many people, it is now inconceivable that you could go without, even though many pain symptoms are insignificant reactions. The long list of possible side effects is ignored, as is the possibility of treating pain using simple household remedies or by making lifestyle changes.

DMSO can be used to treat both chronic and acute pain. After all, it was a popular painkiller in the 1960s. The effect is attributable to the inhibition of nerve conduction to the relevant nerve fibres. It should be noted, however, that pain is a natural warning sign. Just as we criticise the use of the medications mentioned above, we should be aware that these signals can have an important function. When treating sports injuries with DMSO, the swift reduction in pain which DMSO brings about leads to the patient placing too much strain on the affected area too soon, making the original injury worse.

To me, it seems wiser to consider what might be causing the pain and to treat the root problem. It is recognised that headaches, of which there are countless types, can be caused by obstructions in the spine, intolerance to medicines, and diseases of the blood vessels (along with a great number of other possibilities). Once one of these factors has been identified, efforts should be made to treat or avoid it. Painkillers alone will do nothing to cure anything in the long term.

Nevertheless, DMSO, with its wide spectrum of effects, enables us to comprehensively treat a number of painful complaints and diseases. Some examples include tendinitis, intervertebral disc problems, sports injuries, rheumatism, and many more. In addition to relieving pain, the range of pharmacological properties that DMSO offers can treat the root of the disease, often bringing about a cure. Depending on the area causing pain, DMSO can be applied externally in the form of an aqueous solution, taken as a drink, or administered as an infusion. Earache or sinus pain can be treated locally by administering drops of a 25 to 50% DMSO solution. Pain in the oral cavity can be alleviated by swilling the mouth with a DMSO drink solution.

Apart from treating the underlying disease, other measures for treating pain include acupuncture, manual pain therapy, warmth / cold and movement therapy / physiotherapy. Real peppermint oil (Euminz®) is an excellent treatment for many headaches in the forehead or the temples. I am sure we all have our own ways of dealing with a range of different pains, without having to revert to pharmaceutical painkillers.

Dr Morton Walker[19] describes an astonishing case of an 'unintended' cure for pains, involving the disappearance of the kind of phantom pain that can develop following amputations. It is generally thought that these pains cannot be treated directly using medications.

Anna Goldeman, then 65 years old, was suffering from a painful case of bursitis of the right shoulder. Four years previously she had undergone an operation to amputate her left leg at the hip. She had suffered various painful sensations and twitches ever since, as if the removed limb was causing problems. Such sensory phenomena are known as phantom pains and are thought to be caused by neurophysiological reaction patterns. The symptoms can become a source of immense suffering for those affected. Anna Goldeman's bursitis was treated using DMSO and as the pain in her right shoulder disappeared, so did the phantom pain on the other side of her body. The pain never returned. Ten years later, Morton Walker spoke to the doctor who administered the treatment and learned that Anna Goldeman feels just as well now as she did back then. She drew great comfort from the knowledge that DMSO would be able to help her if the dreaded sensations ever returned.

This story illustrates very clearly how DMSO, because of the way it circulates throughout the whole body, can have a holistic, integrated effect even when administered locally.

Pancreatitis

The pancreas, as a secretory organ, is responsible for two extremely important tasks. Firstly, it produces vital metabolic hormones (e.g. insulin) that are released into the bloodstream (endocrine function). Secondly, it produces enzymes that are indispensable in the digestion process; the pancreas sends these enzymes via a central passageway into the first part of the small intestine (exocrine function). These enzymes include substances that help to break down fat and proteins. This is what makes an inflammation in this organ so dangerous. In short, the fundamental problem caused by an inflammation in the pancreatic tissue is the resulting change in the permeability of the enzyme excretory ducts. As a result, the enzymes can become activated too early, causing them to attack the pancreas by digesting itself from within. This can result in the destruction of the adenocytes as well as in an 'enzymatic' attack on and the perforation of other neighbouring abdominal organs. Pancreatitis can occur in an acute or chronic form. There is a range of known causes for inflammation of the pancreas. The most common are gallstones (the pancreatic duct joins the bile duct and both have a common entry into the duodenum), excess consumption of alcohol, and infectious diseases such as mumps or hepatitis. Symptoms include severe pain in the upper abdomen, constipation and fever. DMSO, as an anti-inflammatory agent, can be very useful when treating this condition. There are probably various mechanisms behind its palliative and / or healing effect and they certainly involve DMSO's permeability properties (pervasion, penetrability). It is also possible that DMSO deactivates enzymes directly.

Caution: pancreatitis is a severe illness that often leads to serious complications. It is necessary to abstain from food, to take in large quantities of liquids via infusions from an early stage, and to take painkillers (DMSO also works as a painkiller). Depending on the symptoms and the cause (e.g. infection), additional treatment options such as MMS by infusion should be considered. The advantage of MMS over normal antibiotics and stomach acid inhibitors is that it causes less strain on the body in what is already a critical situation. Due to the acid it contains, I would advise patients suffering from pancreatitis not to take the standard activated MMS solution by mouth. Instead, take ready-to-use CDS (chlorine dioxide solution) products orally, or see my description of the process of preparing pyrogen-free infusions (Chapter 2.5.1). If you want to use DMSO as an anti-inflammatory and pain-relieving medication to treat pancreatitis, you should not administer it in the same infusion as MMS – administer one after the other. Bear in mind that the DMSO infusion can be administered at a relatively fast drop rate, while the oxidative MMS infusion should be administered at a very slow drop rate so that the red blood cells can be loaded steadily with ClO_2.

Parkinson's disease See Neurodegenerative diseases

Polyneuropathy

This term could be translated as 'the disease of many nerves'. As you might expect, it involves a number of very different symptom complexes and a range of possible causes. In general terms, nerve cell and / or nerve fibre damage causes striking and unpleasant sensations, mainly in the extremities. The feet / lower legs or the hands / forearms send signals reporting pain, numbness, prickling and burning sensations. This condition is not always easy to distinguish from restless legs syndrome. The supply of nutrients to the listed areas can become disrupted, resulting in open wounds that heal poorly. Other symptoms include digestive disorders, bladder disorders and restricted pupil reaction.

As already indicated, there is a wide range of causes and the origin of the disease often remains unclear. Polyneuropathy can arise as a result of diabetes, alcoholism, multiple sclerosis, autoimmune diseases, hypothyroidism, medications (chemotherapy) and poisons (lead), vitamin or iron deficiency, infections (Borrelia, glandular fever, HIV, etc.) , cancer, blood vessel inflammations, or it can develop without any identifiable cause. Treatment should initially be focused on the underlying illness if it can be determined. This means that the patient must be weaned off alcohol, must be provided with vitamin supplements, or be treated for diabetes. Furthermore, by using DMSO the damaged nerve cells are given the opportunity to regenerate themselves because of the improved transport of substances to and from the cells. DMSO's anti-inflammatory, pain-relieving and membrane-stabilising effects also help to cure polyneuropathy.

If only the feet and / or hands are affected, treating these areas externally with aqueous DMSO solutions has proven to be effective. Use 60 to 80% preparations, applied with a brush or a spray. In severe cases, DMSO can also be administered internally in parallel with external administration. Starting with a dose of 0.05g per kilogram of body weight, DMSO is administered in the form of diluted drink solutions or infusions, with gradual increases in dose (see Chapter 2).

Case: a few years ago, Mr E. F., 84 years old, felt a burning sensation and an increasing feeling of numbness in both feet. These sensations steadily worsened, with the result that he had to limit the time he spent gardening, which he dearly loved, and he became less confident about driving since using the pedals became increasingly difficult. His doctor took a standard blood test, a neurologist measured his nerve conduction velocity, and he was advised to take alpha-lipoic acid. He was diagnosed with polyneuropathy. There was no noticeable improvement in his condition, and vitamin B injections were tried. It was at about this stage that we spoke for the first time and I suggested taking a more detailed blood test. Conditions such as vitamin deficiencies, thyroid dysfunction, iron deficiency, alcohol misuse, inflammation and many others can be identified very quickly. The man returned to his doctor who then carried out this test but no abnormality was detected. Even though the patient was now suffering from additional symptoms such as sluggishness of the bowels / constipation and low heart frequency, none of the 'usual suspects' could be detected. It was impossible for me to assess the patient more thoroughly since he lived about 150km away. Despite that, the patient tried a few treatments I had recommended, among them the external application of DMSO. This measure effected a significant reduction in symptoms after the first application. The patient was able to garden for longer periods of time and could drive safely again even though the condition had been progressing for a number of years. The symptoms of paraesthesia abated appreciably as a result of this treatment. Since the symptoms return when DMSO treatment is stopped, we can assume that the cause has still not been identified or cured. However, the man is very satisfied with the results he has experienced using DMSO.

Case: Mr B. H., 82 years old, suffered an acute pancreatic inflammation in the spring of 2010. To everyone's surprise he survived this serious illness after a few weeks of treatment in an intensive care ward. However, the pancreas was so badly damaged that it was barely able to produce insulin. That, in turn, led to hugely elevated blood sugar values the patient had become diabetic. He was already describing typical 'phantom sensations' in his feet during the rehabilitation phase and saying, for example, that the nurses should remove his socks even though he was not wearing socks. Soon thereafter he began to suffer severe prickling and burning sensations in his hands. All in all, however, he felt well-cared for by his doctors and he could cope with the symptoms. On my advice he rubbed a DMSO solution onto his hands and, lo and behold, the unpleasant sensations disappeared within minutes. No holistic treatment programme that might have addressed the cause was implemented, neither in the initial stages nor later. Blood sugar values remained dangerously high and the patient had no comprehension of the changes that would be necessary in terms of diet and lifestyle. But he gratefully accepted the relief offered to him by DMSO.

Premenstrual syndrome (PMS)

This condition can involve a number of very different and complex sets of symptoms suffered by many women of childbearing age as a result of a sexual hormone imbalance. Rising and descending levels of these messenger substances in the blood lead to recurring symptoms that mainly affect the emotions and mental performance. Other possible symptoms include pain, changes to the skin, weight fluctuation, digestive complaints and recurring flare-ups of infections and inflammations. DMSO, with its range of balancing and stabilising effects, can be a useful treatment for this set of additional symptoms. Depending on the range of symptoms in each individual case, other treatments can be used to achieve a harmonic balance. Traditionally, phytotherapy, the use of herbs and natural substances, has an important part to play in this regard. Depending on the patient's constitution, preventative measures such as purging, detoxifying, or strengthening can be taken.

DMSO can be taken regularly or sporadically to improve well-being and energy levels. Any three of the methods described in Chapter 2 can be used: application to the skin, drink solution or infusion. An initial dose of 0.05g DMSO per kilogram of body weight is used. For someone weighing 70kg, that would be about 3ml or 1 teaspoon per day.

Prostatitis

This term covers both acute and chronic inflammation of the prostate, as well as the inflammatory and non-inflammatory forms of chronic pelvic pain syndrome. Prostatitis can be caused by bacteria, or it can develop without any indication that such a pathogen is present. Where no evidence of a bacteria can be found, there is a range of possible explanations for the development of the debilitating symptoms, including nerve irritations, autoimmune reactions and muscle tension. Mainstream medical doctors treat bacterial prostatitis using antibiotics. Even when this brings the levels of the bacteria down below the detection threshold, the perceptible symptoms often remain or return (recurrent inflammation). The medicines used to treat the other, non-bacterial form of this disease – alpha-blockers, flavonoids, pollen extracts – also fail to offer a long-term cure, as has been demonstrated in countless clinical trials. Women also have a corresponding tissue structure (female prostate, Skene's gland) that originates from embryonic development. Inflammation can cause very complicated and persistent symptoms here, leading to interstitial cystitis in some cases. However, that is the exact condition for which DMSO has been officially approved as a treatment in the USA.

For these and other reasons, the external or internal administration of DMSO is recommended as a treatment for prostate conditions. Its pain-relieving, anti-inflammatory and regenerative effects make an important contribution to treating both the symptoms and the root cause. It can be applied locally by administering it liberally to the perineum. It can also be drunk or taken as an infusion. If the patient is suffering from a chronic infection, you can try a combination treatment of DMSO and MMS. If myofascial blocks caused by tension are suspected, additional relaxation exercises, stretching or manual pain therapy should be used.

Psoriasis (see also Skin diseases)

This is an inflammatory skin disease that affects the whole body. It can, depending on the extent of the disease, also develop on the nails, joints and organs. It is generally accepted that this is another manifestation of an immune system dysfunction in which the body's cells are attacked, bringing about conditions favourable for an inflammation in the affected area. There are a number of possible causes for the autoimmune reaction. Genetic disposition and previous illnesses can play a role, as can the side effects of medications, nutrition and the psyche. DMSO, as an anti-inflammatory medication that also helps to regulate the immune system, can be used to treat psoriasis. Because the areas of skin affected by the condition can react very sensitively to the substance, I recommend starting external application treatments with highly diluted solutions (e.g. 20% DMSO in purified water). If that is well tolerated the concentration can be increased to the more 'normal' range of between 50 and 75%. The best method is to spray the solution onto the skin once or twice a day. If the joints and / or organs are affected, DMSO can be taken as a drink or as an infusion, either in addition to the external application or instead of it.

Psychosis / anxiety in children See Developmental disorders in children

Pulled muscles See Sports injuries

Respiratory tract infections

These predominantly involve viral and bacterial diseases in the nose, throat and bronchia. In cases of a nasal cold caused by bacteria, drops of a 30 to 40% DMSO solution can be administered and distributed directly into the nostrils using a pipette. Any initial feeling of burning quickly abates and the swelling of the nasal mucosa subsides. In cases of inflamed throat or pharynx, the patient can gargle a similar concentration of DMSO. Bronchitis and lung inflammations are treated systemically: an appropriate solution of DMSO is administered via the skin, as a drink, or by infusion (see Asthma). All infections are treated with a combination of oxidative substances such as MMS, which quickly eliminate the microorganisms causing the problem. Alternating doses of DMSO and MMS (or hydrogen peroxide) has by now become a standard treatment for all kinds of coughs, colds, tonsillitis, etc. among my fellow health practitioners and their friends and families.

Restless legs syndrome (see also Polyneuropathy)

This syndrome is not a 'fashionable' diagnosis or illness as might be suspected from its name. The symptoms were first described more than three hundred years ago. It is one of the most common neurological diseases in society. The condition involves a range of different symptoms but the main ones are a compulsion to move while resting and an associated inability to sleep. In the long term this leads to reduced energy, avolition, forgetfulness, pain, joint problems and depression. It is often very difficult to distinguish this illness from other diseases, some of which can even cause RLS. There are often overlaps or underlying conditions involving hypothyroidism, polyneuropathy, iron deficiency, vitamin B12 deficiency, Parkinson's disease, impaired renal function, chronic infections (Lyme disease), side effects from medications (antidepressants) and more. This often means that many patients spend long and difficult years searching for solutions in the wrong places. Countless appointments with doctors, consultations with various specialists and recurring bouts of the illness are the norm. Some patients suffer so much that they decide to retreat from society, retire early or even resort to suicide. The standard mainstream treatment for these symptoms is Parkinson's medications (L-DOPA, dopamine agonists). Some of these medications have only recently 'won' (post-) approval for this disease, a state of affairs that has been criticised in some quarters and which points to the close association between the pharmaceutical industry and the medical fraternity.60,70 But let us be honest. There are also alternative health practitioners who team up with companies, promote their products in lectures at trade fairs, push their products onto their patients, and are happy to accept the financial rewards. I am convinced that remaining steadfast and honest when offered the opportunity to earn easy money is one of the toughest tests life can throw at us.

Opiates are an alternative treatment option in severe and painful cases of restless legs syndrome. Patients are sometimes given iron and magnesium supplements as well as antiepileptic medications. Some patients only experience mild symptoms, which they are able to manage intuitively using a number of simple measures. These include changing meal times, regulating the sleep–wake cycle, coffee, exercises, hot and cold showers or, very simply, losing weight.

It seems wise to start by searching for the causes. The search might include comprehensive blood tests and looking back at the patient's case history. For example, if there is a suspicion that the illness may be caused by a long-term Lyme disease infection, a different set of holistic measures would be taken than would be the case if renal insufficiency was detected. DMSO can be used as a basic treatment because it works to alleviate symptoms and to cure the root cause. Since, as the name suggests, it is the legs that are affected, it is recommended that you administer DMSO externally onto the legs. In this way you are combining local application (pain relief, relaxant) with internal absorption. Apply aqueous solutions of 60 to 80% DMSO with a brush or a spray bottle to large areas of the skin.

Rheumatism

Rheumatic diseases and symptoms can develop in specific parts of the body (bone, muscle) such as the hands, or they can develop in the body more generally (organs, connective tissue). Rheumatism is a non-specific term describing a wide range of disease processes and conditions; we usually speak of 'rheumatic spectrum disorders' which affect millions of people. The diseases which belong to this category are not uniformly defined and the terms are used differently by different people. This is clearly potentially confusing as this is a field that includes about 450 conditions such as chronic polyarthritis (inflammation in multiple joints), ankylosing spondylitis, psoriatic arthritis, blood vessel inflammations, scleroderma, muscle inflammation (myalgia / myositis) and many others. However, there is general agreement regarding what causes the tissue damage in most cases, namely an imbalance in the immune system. Here too we are discussing the frequently mentioned autoimmune reactions that cause chronic inflammations and damage to tissue. Accordingly, doctors usually prescribe anti-inflammatory medications that suppress the immune system to complement the basic pain-relief medication. However, these medications – cortisone, diclofenac, metamizole and methotrexate – all cause severe side effects when used long-term.

Controlling tissue degeneration, repairing destroyed tissue, relieving pain, improving circulation, regulating the immune system, soothing inflammation; these are all desirable effects that we would hope to acquire from any good anti-rheumatism medication. DMSO gives you all that. That is why DMSO, in its heyday when it was being researched for use as a medication, was intended as a treatment for exactly these kinds of diseases. In his book[19] Morton Walker reports a number of astonishing cases of patients that were cured. Some of these cases are cited below. The quick relief that DMSO can bring to patients suffering from rheumatic joint, muscle and soft tissue diseases is great news for health practitioners and self-users. DMSO can be applied locally or administered systemically as a drink solution or infusion. The appropriate dose depends on the course the disease has taken in each individual case and on how the patient responds to treatment. You will find suggestions in Chapter 2.

Case:[19] Roger Varga, 59 years old, had been suffering from rheumatoid arthritis for a number of years. His whole body, including his spine, was affected. The joint pains had become so severe over the last five years that he was unable to carry on with day-to-day tasks. His wife initiated divorce proceedings because, as Mr Varga says himself, life with him had become unbearable. DMSO infusions brought about an amazing reduction in symptoms within five days and he was able to return to work. Mr Varga repeated the DMSO treatment twice in a period of 14 months and both times he felt excellent afterwards. He applied a 70% DMSO cream locally between the infusion treatments.

Case:[19] Calvin Vernon, 72 years old, was suffering from a combination of rheumatoid arthritis and osteoarthritis (degenerative inflammation of the bone). The symptoms were mainly to be felt in the back, shoulders, hips and left ankle. Mr Vernon underwent a comprehensive five-day treatment that included administering DMSO externally, drinking a solution and taking an infusion. This brought about a significant reduction in joint pain. Walking became easier, his ankle was less swollen and there was increased mobility in every joint. His doctor assessed the patient's condition as being much improved and Mr Vernon stocked up on DMSO to use internally and externally, confident that he would be able to carry on with his work.

In his chapter on arthritis, Morton Walker gives seven other examples of amazing cases that demonstrate the comprehensive healing effect DMSO has in the treatment of this illness. He also stresses that observing a strict diet is just as important for rheumatic patients, as is well known. There are two aspects to a good diet: ensuring you obtain sufficient levels of vitamins and avoiding foods that release large quantities of organic acids when they are digested and metabolised. The foods you eat should be as natural as possible. It would be funny if it wasn't so sad, how some people respond to the advice that they should avoid cheese and sausages. 'What is there left to eat?' they ask mournfully. That is how impoverished our society has become; that is how securely the food industry has us in its grips. We no longer know what treasures nature has provided for us, if only we looked. Even if people do not make the effort to examine what exactly is in their food, simply eating less would be helpful. Evolution has geared the human body towards lack – not abundance! The regulatory circuits of the digestive, metabolic and excretory systems, which have been researched intensively over the last hundred years, prove this. The early stages of any alternative treatment programme for rheumatic diseases should include DMSO administration, detoxification and deacidification measures, and comprehensive advice on diet ... if the patient is open to such changes.

Ringing in the ears See Tinnitus

Scars

Although most people are unaware of this, scars are by no means simply a cosmetic problem. In addition to the fact that they disturb neural pathways close to the surface of the skin, they often cause (via adhesions / degradations) various structural problems and movement limitations. Any knowledgeable orthopaedic shoemaker or physiotherapist will tell you that simple appendicitis or Caesarean scars, as factors causing imbalance, can lead over long periods of time to static interference resulting in joint damage in the feet, knees or hips. These are the physical results of what we generally call interference fields. You do not even need to believe in the theories of acupuncture, the negative effects of surgical scars are so noticeable. Furthermore, in terms of complexity, past injuries cause systemic effects that go way beyond the purely mechanical problems mentioned. Scars in the lower abdomen disturb important meridians and can therefore become chronic fields of interference. Today we know from countless published patient case reports that such interference fields cause severe pain, and that they can be healed. Interference fields can also cause rheumatism, metabolic disorders, fibromyalgia and burnout, not to mention 'easy' complaints such as sleep disorders, lack of energy or nervousness.

So how do we heal scars? There is a range of treatments available, including laser, electrical stimulation and injections. Neural therapy injections are administered using a local anaesthetic such as procaine or lidocaine. The skin is flooded intracutaneously and subcutaneously with a 1 to 2% alkaline solution of the above substances – wheals then fuse together. Since this is scar tissue, the procedure is usually painless. Patients usually notice improvements very quickly. They often report noticeable changes immediately or on the following day, particularly if the scar involved was previously 'active', tended to itch, tingle, or was sensitive to the weather. The method is more effective when combined with DMSO, either as a mixture or with DMSO applied to the skin beforehand, followed by the injection. The reasons for this were explained in detail in Chapter 2.5.2.

Along with this standard scar treatment to resolve the interference, which is usually only administered once or twice at the most, continuing with repeated applications of DMSO over the long term is advisable. The enzymatic effects of the liquid in terms of improving the condition

ot the tissue were described in the section on 'Pharmacological properties'. Improving the condition of low-grade scar tissue through patient,
external application of DMSO is an amazing opportunity to repair the
function and the appearance of the affected areas of skin. You need do
nothing more than dab the scar regularly with a 60 to 75% DMSO solution once a day and allow this to be absorbed as completely as possible. If the area of skin is very small you can use a wad of cotton wool.
If the affected area is larger, using a baking brush or a spray bottle may
be more appropriate. In some cases scars can be made to 'disappear'
completely using other measures that are easy to carry out.

Case: S. H., female, 14 years old, was born with a missing calf bone
(fibula). This developmental defect is known by the name fibular aplasia
and is usually accompanied by a shortening of the upper and / or lower
leg. Consequently, those affected must undergo a series of operations
in their childhood and teenage years if they are to have any chance of
being able to walk normally. These operations leave extensive scarring.
Along with the common mechanisms of interference which surgical
scars cause simply because of the traces of talcum powder present on
surgical gloves, this is also a serious cosmetic problem for patients. We
got to know the girl, her sister and her mother in Italy. A friendship developed between us and we would meet once a year. The extensive surgical scars on her right leg were hardened and made a disturbing impression. Because S. had become terrified of syringes, she adamantly
rejected my suggestion that we wheal the scar. However, she did agree
to have a 75% DMSO solution applied to the scar and she quickly became accustomed to the initial feeling of itching and tingling. She has
been using DMSO 'on and off' for six months now and reports that the
scar tissue is constantly improving. Since she still has one operation to
undergo, which will hopefully be her last, she has the opportunity to
prepare the skin on this area in advance and to treat it effectively
afterwards.

Case: Mr H. F., 45 years old, suffered an open fracture of the thigh bone
in a motorbike accident in 1982. A metal plate and nine screws were
implanted, making a second operation necessary at a later point to remove these materials. This left a 28cm scar on the outer side of the left
thigh and various adhesions had formed here. Almost thirty years later,
after applying DMSO externally only three times, there have been visible

and perceptible improvements to the tissue. Encouraged by this Mr F. intends to continue to treat the scar with DMSO, perhaps using it in combination with procaine / lidocaine and hydrogen peroxide.

Sciatica (see also Back / intervertebral disc problems)

A number of different symptoms and their causes are bundled together under the term 'sciatica'. Serious irritation or damage at the root of the sciatic nerve is usually accompanied by symptoms of deficiency and / or pains that reach all the way into the legs. Lumbago, damage to the body of the vertebra, osteoporosis, (bone) tumours and even deep-lying shingles can all lead to severe back pain that is often called 'sciatica' by patients. Pain in the area of the lumbar vertebra and the sacrum must therefore be examined very carefully. The focus of the treatment, following the diagnosis, should be on the root cause. In this regard DMSO can be a very useful basic treatment. The symptoms often quickly improve when a 60 to 75% solution is applied locally over an extensive area. Internal administration as a drink or infusion can amplify the effect even further. Only qualified and experienced doctors and alternative health practitioners should administer intramuscular injections containing a mixture of DMSO (20%) and a local anaesthetic. A series of such injections into the affected muscle groups can be administered over a period of 3 to 5 days.

Scleroderma See Rheumatism

Shingles / herpes zoster

Shingles is actually caused by the reactivation of the varicella zoster virus which continues to linger dormant in the spinal marrow and / or cranial nerve ganglia for a lifetime after initial infection with chickenpox. Close to 100% of the population carry the virus, even if the initial infection ran its course without symptoms. Further proliferation of the virus can occur when the immune system is weakened by stress, chemotherapy or by a host of other factors. The risk of shingles rises with age because immunity decreases as we become older. The main symptoms are severe pains and the formation of inflamed rashes / blisters on the skin along the area supplied by the affected nerves. Even though these symptoms are agonizing, the real danger of this illness is posed by the complications that can subsequently arise. Up to about a quarter of all those affected develop symptoms that can remain for a long time after the skin problems have disappeared. The most common of these is post-zoster neuralgia which involves severe and chronic nerve pain as well as symptoms of paralysis.

Dr Morton Walker[19] describes the case of a 66-year-old woman who was suffering from shingles in the oral cavity. That can occur when cerebral nerves are affected by the infection. The patient was diagnosed by her dentist, whose advice she had sought because of the severe pain in the mouth. She was not ready to accept that there was nothing the medical profession could do to help her so, on her own initiative, she treated herself using a DMSO solution. She always had DMSO with her as a first aid measure and she prepared a 50% solution. On the first day she used that 3 times as a mouthwash and to cleanse the throat. She repeated this on the second day but combined the DMSO with aloe vera because of irritation to the mucosa. After just two days the blisters had disappeared, and they have never returned.

Dr Walker describes a clinical study carried out by Dr William Campbell Douglas in 1971 in which 46 shingles patients were treated externally with DMSO: 50 to 90% DMSO solutions were applied directly to the areas of affected skin. It became clear that DMSO, when applied at a very early stage, could shorten the duration of the illness and reduce the risk of complications significantly.

According to Dr Walker the researchers were also successful in treating herpes zoster and herpes simplex using a mixture of DMSO and vitamin C.

Shoulder–arm syndrome / frozen shoulder

(see also Pains, Sports injuries)

These terms are used to describe a number of different pain syndromes along the cervical spine / shoulder / arm axis. The number of different causes is even greater than the number of specific forms in which they can manifest themselves, which means that matters often end in diagnostic and therapeutic chaos. Patients find themselves going from one clinic to the next, a journey that often comes to be viewed as a personal odyssey. When one of these patients arrives at my clinic, I often hear such things as 'After noticing the first symptoms I waited far too long before doing anything', or 'I don't understand why nothing seems to help.' Morton Walker emphasises that the shoulder joint and the physical structures linked to it respond well to topical DMSO treatment. Even when diagnostic imaging techniques show an accumulation of deposits, DMSO can be relied on to wield its regenerative effects. Physical therapy measures should always be geared towards expanding the space in the shoulder joint. It can be assumed that the severe pains are caused in full or in part by a shortening of the respective muscles and their tendons. Often, the shoulder joint itself is sound and the movement limitations in the shoulder are actually caused by transferred pain from the cervical spine and the hardening of the musculature that results. It is also possible for the structural chain of the skeleton, nerves and muscles to transfer pain from the cervical spine and shoulder into the elbow, the wrist or the hand, or vice versa. This sometimes (perhaps quite often) leads to rash diagnoses of carpal tunnel syndrome, and to patients going under the knife unnecessarily.

First the word, then the plant, and lastly the knife.
Asclepius

Case: Mr M. R., 47 years old, had been suffering from severe shoulder pains for over 6 months and movement in his left arm was badly restricted. A lorry driver by trade, he was no longer able to complete the tasks that his work demanded of him even though he was taking painkillers by the gram. He was on official sick leave and appeared quite desperate for relief, although he would not admit it. As a result of some artful persuasion by his friends (or threats, as I later discovered), he found himself in my practice and we began by treating the whole shoulder with a topical administration of a 75% DMSO solution. We also injected a mixture containing a local anaesthetic and some other ingredients into specific areas of the skin associated with important pain points. Manual pain therapy (myofascial treatment following the Golgi method) did not yield any significant results. The patient was ambivalent regarding the tuina method (Chinese massage). I gave him some homework in the form of the 'elephant's trunk' exercise (a favourite with children), and another exercise which stretches the joints in the opposite direction. I told Mr R. to spend a few minutes every day holding a bucket filled with water in his left hand with the shoulder completely relaxed (painless) as a way of relieving pressure on the joint when the shoulder is moved forward. When he returned for his second appointment, M. R. brought some good news with him. The range of movement had increased and the pain had decreased – he was no longer taking painkillers. However, after such a long time, the problem was very compli-

cated and the pain, as was to be expected, was being referred to a different area, in this case to the front musculature of the upper arm. We were
not discouraged by this and we gamely continued to brush DMSO onto
a large area of the skin. We continued with the intracutaneous injections
at important points, and with the tuina treatment. The patient showed
me how he did the exercises and I corrected the movements where
necessary. He reported that he found the bucket exercise very beneficial.
This was repeated at the third appointment. The patient reported that
some muscle pain remained when using the biceps. We agreed that he
would continue with the exercises for a further five days and that we
would administer a DMSO infusion at the next appointment. We even
searched for a good vein. But Plan B was not necessary. M. R. told me
shortly afterwards that he wanted to return to work because the pain
had disappeared. Friends of his told me a couple of weeks later that he
had been helping them with some strenuous building work in his spare
time. Four months have passed since then and the shoulder can now
tolerate the whole range of movements and physical strain without pain.
Every now and again M. R. enjoys telling me about people from his
social circle who have undergone joint operations.

Sinusitis

This condition appears to have become a 'national disease'. It involves
acute or chronic inflammations in the four symmetrically paired cavities
around the nose: the frontal sinus, the sphenoid sinus, the ethmoid sinus
and the maxillary sinus. The disease is usually caused by a virus, bacteria
or an allergic reaction, which leads to swelling in the mucous membrane
of the sinuses. The mucus produced in these cavities is obstructed, leading in turn to a purulent site. DMSO can be used to combat both the
causes and the symptoms simultaneously. It has an antibacterial and an
anti-allergenic effect. It reduces swelling of the mucous membrane and
promotes the regeneration of inflamed tissue. Drops of a 25 to 40%
aqueous solution is administered directly into the nostrils (2 to 3 drops
each side). At first, the vasodilatory effect can be very forceful and may
cause severe itching or burning sensations for a few seconds or minutes.
Often, that happens because the drops run too far, reaching the throat.
If that is the case, you can relieve the sensations by drinking water. Within a few minutes patients usually feel pleasant sensations as the sinuses
open and the pains subside. How often you should administer this treatment depends on how the condition develops. These days I use DMSO

nose and ear drops to treat all inflammatory diseases in this area. I am always impressed by how quickly patients recover.

Case: I personally suffered a bout of sinusitis in June 2012. The blocked nose, difficulty in swallowing, facial pain, burning forehead, shivering and fatigue all came out of the blue, so we can assume it was a viral infection. The previous day was Seven Sleepers Day and the weather had not exactly been summerlike. I gave myself a high-dose ascorbic acid infusion and drank an improvised 'alchemistic' cocktail of right-turning lactic acid, barley grass powder, alkaline salts and a few other ingredients. The infusion brought back the warmth and energy into my body, but the face and jaw pain and the swallowing difficulties disturbed my sleep. Eventually it occurred to me to try my frequently recommended DMSO drops, so I tilted my head backwards and put some 40% solution into each nostril. To distribute the liquid I closed the nostrils by pressing against the sides of the nose with my thumb and forefinger and built up some pressure. I immediately felt a warm burning sensation, which soon disappeared. Subsequently my nose was clear again and the pain quickly subsided. I repeated this the next morning and was able to go about my normal working day.

Why did I not resort to using MMS in this situation? I had heard that high doses of ascorbic acid have a pro-oxidative effect. I wanted to try that out. However, there is a great difference between the cost of the two treatments. A dose of MMS costs just a few pennies. In contrast, a 15 gram ascorbic acid infusion costs about £22 simply for the product. But the latter has a number of additional positive regeneration effects and I was keen to give myself a treat.

Skin ageing See Ageing

Skin diseases

So-called 'skin efflorescence' or rashes – i.e. patches of skin that are noticeably different from healthy skin – can develop of their own accord, or as a result of other underlying diseases, including atopic eczema, psoriasis, fungal infections, and childhood diseases. Furthermore, skin conditions can be inflammatory, painful, or itchy. As an anti-inflammatory, anti-allergenic, pain-relieving agent, an appropriate solution of DMSO can be applied externally to great effect. The best way in which to administer the treatment is by dabbing or spraying the substance onto the skin. How often the treatment should be repeated depends on the progression of the disease in each individual case. In many cases, DMSO soothes the itching, pain, inflammation or the tension within an hour, reducing the risk of a secondary bacterial or fungal infection.

Case: Ms C. O., 55 years old, suddenly found her torso and arms covered in a number of red, inflamed, and open lesions. She suffered severe pain and itching that kept her awake at night. The case initially puzzled the attending physician. After a comprehensive investigation, the patient was diagnosed with soft-tissue rheumatism (reactive perforating collagenosis). Patients with a diabetic metabolic condition and elevated uric acid levels are susceptible to such extreme elimination reactions, which can be understood to be the detoxifying response of a body carrying a heavy toxic load. She asked me for advice because she was not satisfied with the effect of the various creams she had been prescribed. We immediately began treatment by dabbing the numerous pustules with a 70% DMSO solution. She told me the next day that she had finally been able to sleep on the previous night. She has now been using DMSO intermittently for three months because she is still seeing progress as the severely damaged skin repairs and regenerates itself. DMSO will help to avoid scarring as the skin heals. The patient has gradually implemented the suggestions I made regarding step-by-step changes to her diet and she has taken detoxifying measures to hopefully avoid further escalations of this type in future.

Case: L. S., 8 years old, had fungal infections the size of my palm on his lower leg. His mother had initially tried fungal infection creams but could not keep the infection in check in the long term. She was also not keen to use such substances every day and over a long period of time. She tried using a 75% DMSO solution which she brushed onto the boy's legs. She had her doubts regarding the treatment because of the initial reaction whereby the skin becomes red. But she trusted her gut instinct and repeated the treatment a further two times. The fungal skin infection disappeared without trace.

Skin ulcers See Wounds

Spinal cord injuries

Injuries to the spinal cord do not only sound dangerous, but the paralysis that can arise as a result is, in many cases, irreversible. Depending on the extent of the injuries to the nerve fibres in the affected area, the neurological dysfunction can recede if the swelling to the injured tissue that develops at the same time does not exert too much pressure on the nerve fibres for too long. The diameter of the spinal canal is fixed by the natural 'protective tube' formed by the spaces in the vertebrae. The nerve fibres have no room for manoeuvre. You will be familiar enough with the effect after reading the section on back and intervertebral disc problems. The first priority with regard to any traumatic injury to the central nervous system is to ease the pressure. If, for example, someone has a fall and sustains a head injury causing internal bleeding, the pressure is relieved by drilling the skull. The blood can then flow out of this hole, easing the pressure inside the rigid bone of the skull. Such a procedure is obviously of no use when an influx of fluid swells the tissue as a result of a spinal cord injury. DMSO can accomplish great things in such cases. When administered early enough, it quickly alleviates the swelling and supports the regeneration of the nerve function. This is illustrated beautifully in the case of a certain patient described by Morton Walker in his book.[19]

On 15 September 1979, Clara Fox from Washington state was shocked and stunned when she learned that her son Bill had had a near-fatal accident and was now completely paralysed. Fortunately, within a few hours of the accident, he was transferred to a hospital where Dr George Greccos was working in the intensive care unit. During the first ten days following Bill's devastating accident, Dr Greccos treated him holistically using DMSO infusions. Bill had broken his neck above the fifth cervical vertebra and was completely paralysed from that point down. He lay there, head shorn, with the ugly steel tongs used to stabilise his spine penetrating his skull. Ropes and pulleys with weights fixed the position of his neck at the crucial point to give it the best chance of recovery. He remained in traction for a further 45 days after leaving the intensive care ward, where he had been lying for four days, teetering between life and death. In total, he spent more than six months in hospital. Bill was first given DMSO seven hours after the accident. Back then it was assumed that DMSO had to be administered within 90 minutes in cases of injuries to the spinal cord or stroke, if at all possible. After a few days of treatment he could feel sensations, first in the shoulders and arms, then in the upper chest. His family was overjoyed. By the end of his DMSO treatment he had regained normal bladder function. It was a phenomenal recovery and Dr Greccos remembers explaining to the parents in the first conversation he had with them that it was unlikely that their son would survive, so serious were the injuries shown by the x-ray. Should he survive, he would be permanently paralysed. The doctor realised that DMSO had literally saved Bill's life by drawing the fluids, and thereby the pressure, from the spinal cord and head. It also helped Bill regain feeling in his body. Without DMSO, Bill would have died. Five weeks after discontinuing DMSO treatment, an operation was carried out to repair damaged cartilage. Two stainless steel rods were implanted and fused together using bone and muscle tissue from Bill's hip. The operation was successful. He was then put on a physical therapy programme as part of the rehabilitation process. However, postoperative pain prevented him from taking part, and he lacked the motivation and enthusiasm necessary to overcome this hurdle. Over time his condition deteriorated and he and his mother felt that it was necessary to restart taking DMSO infusions. Hospital staff would only allow him some topical applications, which minimised the pain in certain parts of his body. After a while, Bill's family noticed smooth and fluid motion in Bill's legs as they applied DMSO. The hospital staff did not take the descriptions of these movements seriously until Dr Greccos saw this movement one day as he was talking to Bill. He came out of the room amazed and awestruck, saying that he now knew what the family had been expressing. By that point the family had been campaigning for three months to restart infusion treatment but with no success. Now, shortly after the Christmas holidays, their wish was granted, but on certain conditions. Bill would first have to undergo a number of neurological tests at a specialist hospital. If these tests indicated that there was hope of further improvement, more tests would be carried out twice weekly to assess any developments made during the course of the recently approved DMSO treatment. If the tests did not indicate any significant changes, DMSO treatment would be discontinued. Bill's condition improved quickly and continuously from that day on. He could now tolerate the maximum physical therapy for three to five hours a day without pain and he only showed signs of exhaustion because he worked so hard. The musculature of his arms recovered and he was proud of his biceps. On 13 March 1980, the previous neurological test results were re-evaluated. They were astounding: all readings indicated dramatic improvement. In addition, feeling was returning to his right foot. He returned home and was able to eat, brush his teeth, shave, comb his hair, get dressed and bathe, all by himself. Just six months previously, his family had been getting accustomed to the idea that he would be completely paralysed for the remainder of his life. Now, he was able to operate his wheelchair with precision.

Bill's mother later wrote a letter to a political representative: 'During the last six months, I have spent many hours in Dr Jacob's clinic with his beautiful and caring staff, watching miracle after miracle take place directly before my eyes. I have seen people who have been totally paralysed for twenty years or more being treated and starting to move. The wonder in their eyes is indeed a sight to behold. I have witnessed the awe in the eyes and actions of a young couple whose child is being treated for Down's syndrome, and listened with rapt attention as they relate how far that child has come from death's door to his present condition. I have sent or personally brought people with various illnesses or pains to Dr Jacob's clinic and seen them smile with the utmost satisfaction at having been cured or helped after years of discomfort and pain. And then I have sat back and watched Dr Jacob, absolutely ecstatic, after another successful treatment. How very proud and happy he is to be able to help this human race of ours. I have also done a lot of reading and research into the full and real story of this remarkable drug, and I can only summarize all my hopes and prayers, along with millions of others, that this humble man can see all his work and dreams materialize into that final success of having DMSO returned to the market by the Federal Drug Administration*, so that all Americans might have the opportunity to be helped or saved through those efforts. I urge everyone who is connected with this prospect: please check all the facts carefully, and help to answer these prayers.'

Spinal stenosis

This condition involves a constriction in the free lumen of the spinal canal, at the point where the spinal cord or its branches are to be found. According to various statistical studies, almost a quarter of those over 60 are affected. Caused by an enlargement of the facet joints and / or the ligamenta flava that connect adjacent vertebrae, the diameter of the spinal canal can be reduced by up to 1.5cm. You can gain an understanding of that by making a hole with your thumb and forefinger, and then making that hole smaller and smaller by increasingly bending the

* News: As of November 2015 DMSO ampules are officially available in Germany!

221

forefinger. It is only logical that that cannot be good for the nerve fibres within, neither in terms of their function nor in terms of the blood supply via the vessels. Since it is usually the lumbar area that is affected, the result is back pain and dysfunction of the legs after exertion.

I believe that the mainstream medical establishment is taking the easy way out when explaining the cause of these symptoms. It opts for the comfortable, age-old argument that this kind of degeneration is inevitable in *Homo sapiens* considering the fact that we walk upright on two legs and that we now, in the modern age, live to such old age. However, perhaps we should be asking ourselves whether daily habits common to our society, which we proudly describe as being civilised and highly advanced, might be making a contribution to the large number of people who develop spinal canal constrictions. These habits include spending long periods in unbalanced postures at work or when driving or watching television, unnatural breathing, poor nutrition, and preventing detoxification and regeneration processes.

Sooner or later, patients are usually given an MRI scan to obtain an image of the structure and condition of the spinal canal. The treatment most commonly offered is surgery with decompression and / or stabilisation (brace). The number of operations carried out, operations which are often played down and described as being 'minimally invasive', has multiplied over the last few decades. As a result, a Gold Rush spirit has broken out among orthopaedic surgeons and neurosurgeons, and outpatient surgical clinics shoot up out of the ground like mushrooms. This is a further example of how certain 'experts' draw significant sums of money from the system, all at the public's expense. Instead of striving for a natural lifestyle and utilising simple treatment methods (household remedies), it has become very fashionable to have a back operation. The long-term consequences for health, and the financial burden on the system, are considerable. The surgeons I know enjoy driving around in luxury cars …

Incidentally, spinal canal stenosis is also common in (riding) horses and that trend is increasing. This is the result of poor riding style, overworking the horses, incorrectly fitting saddles, etc.

When I first became familiar with DMSO I admit that I did not really believe that doctors and vets could use it to treat spinal stenosis successfully. I had too much respect for this disease and perhaps I was captive to the widespread belief that surgery is the only option. But then in September 2012 I met Ms Maier …

Case: Ms M. Meier, 83 years old, had been a hard-working woman all her life. After all, her husband had lost a leg in the war. He had been conscripted as a sixteen-year-old in March 1944 and sent as cannon fodder to fight the futile battles on the Eastern Front. I remember this detail because my father suffered the same fate as a sixteen-year-old the following winter, spending months in a field hospital before returning home as one of the seriously wounded. Even in those last days of the insanity, decorations for bravery were handed out with zeal to these traumatised children – a betrayed generation! 'War always begins with a lie' is a phrase that has remained with me ever since. Ms Meier worked hard and overcame some significant hurdles. Now, however, it was her husband who called my colleague Karin Fietzner, asking her with great agitation for some speedy assistance. Ms Meier had been using a rollator walking aid for a long while, but now the pain was so severe that she was at a complete loss as to what to do. Her back was causing her enormous pain and her right leg often gave way at the knee, causing her to fall to the ground. The knee itself was very painful. It became apparent that she was taking 100mg of aspirin every day so I was not surprised to discover that the falls caused a formidable effusion of blood. Fortunately she had not fractured any bones. She told me that she was taking cortisone tablets every day and that she suffered from spinal stenosis and arthrosis of the knee. She suffered symptoms of lymph accumulation and lymphoedema in the arms and legs as a result of a breast operation that involved the removal of the lymph nodes.

After extensive physical therapy, she asked us for other treatment options so we told her about DMSO's natural regenerative properties. She was immediately very keen and there was no turning back. To cut a long story short, Ms Meier responded wonderfully to DMSO. After the first infusion she was able to get up from the treatment table much more gracefully – the pain had receded. After the second infusion she gave me her rollator and aimed purposefully towards the stairs. I jumped after her to support her because she had not realised that her muscles would need some time to catch up with the sense of euphoria she felt. After the fourth infusion she reported a significant reduction in the circumference of her arms and legs. The 'pillow' on the back of her hand had disappeared and her watch hung loosely on her wrist. She was now ready to discuss discontinuing the cortisone and she reduced the daily dose of aspirin. This was important because it was clear that the cortisone was damaging the tissue and it was difficult to find a footing for the infusion needle in the 'papery' skin. The high doses of aspirin she had been taking regularly caused unwanted bleeding.

Now, after the sixth infusion, Ms Meier is even more excited (as, indeed, are we). The pain in the knees has disappeared and the condition of her blood vessels has improved considerably. The oedemas have continued to reduce significantly. As she was leaving the treatment room one day, she crossed paths with a patient from Hannover who was here for the first time and who had never seen her before. He looked at Ms Meier with curiosity and said, 'Oh, that is a radiant face, like a fresh apple!' Everyone who was there agreed and Ms Meier seemed to grow a few inches with pride. She can now walk confidently and briskly. She has forgotten the sense of despair that she felt when we first got to know one another just a few weeks ago. One can feel that she dreads the moment we tell her she no longer needs further infusions, but that moment will soon arrive.

What do you think the cost difference between DMSO, on the one hand, and a purely symptomatic cortisone treatment and / or surgery on the spine, on the other hand, might be? The cost of mainstream medical treatment is, of course, significantly higher than the cost of the treatment that cured Ms Meier. But no one seems to be asking this question! If you do not have the officially approved authorisation, and are not working within the medical mainstream and its associated traditions, you cannot expect the authorities to absorb the cost of treatment. An upside down state of affairs, ignorance, mismanagement – whatever you think of the rigid bureaucracy of the health system, vain doctors, greedy pharmaceutical and medical technology companies, or of the politicians responsible for health strategy, there is a solution!

If you turn your back on the stipulations and 'prescriptions' of the mainstream approach, it is possible to find a path that will really lead you towards good health. You have an opportunity to use alternative and natural medicine consciously and thoughtfully – all the while avoiding the unnecessary health insurance supplementary tariffs that are widely advertised (in Germany), vaccination recommendations (there are no forced vaccinations!), or so-called screening programmes. As a responsible and well-informed patient, you can consciously decide to change your lifestyle and your spending habits, and pay for diagnosis, treatment or educational costs from your own pocket. By making this carefully considered decision, you become a private patient in the true sense of the word – totally independent and uninfluenced by the patronising ways of legislative health authorities and medical insurance companies.

Sports injuries

This is one of the main fields of application for DMSO, which is mainly known for the way it supports the regeneration of tissue. In my experience this category includes bruises, strains and sprains. Chronic complaints resulting from repeated overstraining of particular parts of the body, or from recurring inflammations, also belong to this category. And we should not forget fractured bones. These require urgent medical or surgical attention, but it is often helpful to give additional treatment using DMSO beforehand and afterwards. In all these cases, DMSO is used first and foremost to limit or to alleviate swelling, pain, haematomas and inflammations. That is why it is so important to brush or spray the affected area with DMSO as soon as possible after suffering injury.

The dose of DMSO used varies depending on the location of the injury. For injuries below the waistline, 70 to 90% preparations can normally be applied immediately. Lower doses should be used to treat injuries located above the waistline, particularly on the face and head (start with a 60% solution in such cases). Refer to the images and advice given in Chapter 2.2 regarding external application. It is important to allow the DMSO to be completely absorbed or washed off before clothing is worn. In severe cases, mixtures of DMSO and diclofenac (e.g. Diclac®, Voltaren® gel) can be used to achieve a stronger anti-inflammatory and pain-relieving effect. However, this mixture should only be used once every two to three days, otherwise it can damage the skin.

Morton Walker[19] writes about the effectiveness of DMSO bandages. An appropriate bandage is soaked in DMSO solution and wrapped around the affected body part. A waterproof bandage (or cling film) is then wrapped around the bandage, so that as much DMSO as possible can be absorbed by the tissue over a long period of time.

Morton Walker describes numerous examples of sports injuries healed using DMSO. A number of people known to me have used DMSO solutions to treat joint and soft tissue injuries, almost all of whom have experienced very positive results. DMSO is always a 'safe bet' when treating these types of injuries (the same is true for arthritic and rheumatic conditions). You can look forward to success as you are carrying out the treatment. I would like to give one example here. My wife suffered a serious knee injury during the obligatory school skiing trip over 25 years ago. Back then in the early 1980s the injury was not examined, diagnosed or treated. We can assume that the meniscus and the capsule were damaged. Since then she has regularly suffered from severe recurring pains and limited movement – until recently. After finally hitting upon the idea of treating this old joint injury externally with DMSO, the knee joint is now (after two applications) practically back to normal and it can bear the full weight of the body.

Morton Walker[19] writes about a survey, carried out in the spring of 1980, of 39 professional sports medics who were questioned regarding their use of DMSO. Because these doctors were responsible for medical supervision at professional sports clubs, and because knowledge of the therapeutic possibilities of DMSO was already carefully guarded even back then, only seven doctors indicated that they used the substance. They said that they used it to treat inflamed joints, sprains, swelling, tendinitis, bursitis, muscle bruising and gout. The only side effects reported were bad breath and the temporary local redness of skin when administering external treatment. Walker describes the case of the Atlanta Falcons' former running back, Haskel Stanback, who, in 1978, sprained his ankle during his first game after being named as a regular starter for the season. The x-ray showed a chipped bone and torn ligaments. His big opportunity was blown. The team managers told him to take his padding home. But someone gave Stanback a bottle of DMSO and told him to apply it to his ankle once every hour, even through the night. He returned to the club that Monday without any swelling in his ankle. The doctors said they would wait until Wednesday before deciding whether he was fit to play because the team had Tuesday off. So Stanback continued to take DMSO for a further two days. He was present at the training session on Wednesday and was able to walk, run, tackle and throw the ball – everything you would expect a professional American football player to be able to do. The following Sunday he was on the pitch playing once more. Being able to play is the most important thing for sportspeople. According to Stanback's doctor, DMSO improves healing and decreases the rest time required before returning to the field following an injury.

Stroke See Infarctions

Sunburn

Redness and burning sensations on the skin are signals that an inflammatory reaction is underway and that a prolonged process of tissue repair will be necessary. DMSO has a pain-relieving, anti-inflammatory and regenerative effect. Areas of skin affected by sunburn should be sprayed finely with a 30 to 60% DMSO solution. This can be repeated 3 to 5 hours later, as necessary.

Caution: if the patient had applied a synthetic sunscreen beforehand (not ideal because of the toxins they contain), this should be washed off as thoroughly as possible before applying DMSO. Use only water and, if necessary, a pure soap – no shower gels etc.

The concentration of DMSO can be increased up to 75% and this can be used until the skin has completely recovered. In acute cases, DMSO can be combined with MMS or hydrogen peroxide solutions with great results. MMS is not activated in this method, but is sprayed undiluted directly onto the skin and washed away thoroughly with water after 30 seconds. Unactivated MMS has a very alkaline pH value that helps to soothe the damaged skin. However, in the case of sunburn the old adage is true: prevention is better than cure! And by that I do not mean coating yourself with huge quantities of the cosmetic industry's chemical cocktails. Appropriate, protective clothing and / or staying in (partially) shadowed areas are still the best measures by which to prevent sunburn, even though that solution might be free of charge and 'uncool'. The skin, immune system and detoxification organs often groan under the burden placed on them by the use of commercial sunscreens and other cosmetics, deodorants and hairsprays. Simply reading the list of ingredients gives the impression that the product is a long way away from being what we would describe as 'natural'. However, we humans really are a 'natural product' and we should, therefore, use substances that are as natural as possible.

Tendinitis

It is vital that the connective tissue that holds us together is in good condition if we are to have a complete and natural range of movement and harmonious control over our musculoskeletal system. When you discuss with young medical students their first experiences of dissecting a corpse, they often report with astonishment the visual impact of seeing the muscle fascia and the tendons that connect the muscles to bones. These supporting structures, which are often mistakenly thought to be passive, actually work together in harmony throughout the whole body, constantly communicating with one another while we sit, stand, walk and run. That is why a disease in one area of connective tissue can, in the long term, lead to inappropriate weight bearing, incorrect posture and resulting damage to the skeleton. Often when someone complains of tennis elbow (which, incidentally, is rarely because of playing tennis) we might be tempted to think that they are exaggerating. However, the suffering caused by the chain reaction initially triggered by local inflammation is often immense. Patients adopt relieving postures, become afraid of physical work and find it impossible to sleep. DMSO can come to the rescue – quickly! And all without cortisone, operations or the long-term use of painkillers.

There are overlaps here with the section on 'Sports injuries' because excess or traumatic strain on the musculoskeletal system often tends to cause inflammations. The true cause of (chronic) tendinitis can also be incorrect or repetitive movement patterns, bad quality shoes, pressure, infection, rheumatic reactions, and many other reasons. Such factors will need to be dealt with if you wish to treat the root cause and achieve a real cure. I have often seen how such a simple measure as walking barefoot at home has quickly healed chronic tendinitis. This is another excellent example of why our habits should be oriented around what evolution had in mind for us.

DMSO is usually administered externally, directly onto the physical structures affected. These areas of the body, which are usually close to joints, are brushed or sprayed with generous amounts of the aqueous DMSO solution. Allow plenty of time for the DMSO to be absorbed through the skin and to reach the site of the inflammation before getting dressed (about 15 to 20 minutes).

Tennis elbow / golfer's elbow See Tendinitis

Thrombosis (tendency)

A tendency towards excessive blood coagulation can be genetic in origin or can be developed later in life. Taking the contraceptive pill from an early age and smoking are both factors that greatly increase the risk of thrombosis. Elevated blood pressure, metabolic diseases, renal dysfunction and other heart and circulation problems can also cause imbalances in the coagulation system and increase aggregation. There is then a risk of developing an embolism. These at-risk patients are often given 'blanket' prescriptions of well-known anticoagulants that are propagated by the pharmaceutical industry and obediently pre-scribed by the medical fraternity. Only now are we gradually hearing critical voices increasingly clearly, pointing out the serious problems that arise as a result of taking these medications over long periods of time.

In my opinion this is a typical example of how the real cause of a disease, in this case the risk of thrombosis (with the exception of the genetic form), is covered up and ignored. Instead of explaining to patients how their suboptimal diets and lifestyle choices are affecting their health, and giving them appropriate 'homework', they are put on drugs, often for the remainder of their lives, that will only have a super-ficial effect. This is the perfect business model; someone somewhere is cashing in and no one is raising any objections. Not even the health in-surance companies. The business risk is zero for the pharmaceutical companies because they are attracting customers that are fully depend-ent on their products. This kind of mass-produced product sold to hordes of badly misinformed patients is described internally as a 'cash cow'.

First of all, we should be clear that an individual's risk of developing a thrombus can be drastically reduced by making targeted lifestyle changes. Avoiding hormone pills and giving up nicotine are vitally important steps. While you will have to do your own research regarding alternative means of contraception, we can help you in your efforts to give up smok-ing. It is also important to take measures to keep the blood vessels healthy. That can include simple things such as drinking plenty of water, taking exercise, and limiting the amount of sugar, 'bad' fats, milk and meat that you eat.

I can hear some of you say: 'That is all well and good but what will help when the patient has already developed arteriosclerosis, or a heart valve dysfunction, or renal deficiency or a number of other diseases? These illnesses are not exclusively the result of incorrect lifestyle choices, they can also be caused by infections or accidents.' You would, of course, be correct in saying that. That is why it is important to discover, in each individual case, to what extent it is possible to treat the disease at its root cause. By using DMSO, there is the opportunity of both reducing coagulation directly, and of having a regenerative effect on the affected physiological functions. To achieve these effects it is necessary to get a sufficiently high quantity of the substance into the blood. It is possible to achieve that by using any of the three methods familiar to us: cutane-ous absorption, drink solution and infusion. For advice, dilution recommendations and total daily doses, see Chapter 2. The duration of treatment is based on how the condition develops.

Tic douloureux See Neuralgias

Tinnitus

Tinnitus (ringing in the ears) is a very common problem that can cause enormous suffering. It is still not known exactly what causes the condition and, as a result, no standard treatment has been developed. It appears that there are no reliable clinical trials based on statistically meaningful patient numbers to support any tinnitus treatments, be they from the mainstream or alternative medicine camps. This is naturally attributable to the fact that the causes and triggers vary greatly from patient to patient. These can include impacted wax, infections / inflammations of the outer or middle ear, otosclerosis (disease of the bone near the middle ear), Lyme disease, chronic and acute exposure to loud noises, hearing impairment and hearing loss, Ménière's disease, acoustic neuroma, autoimmune reactions, etc.

It is often thought that the disease is caused both by a circulation and supply deficiency to the structures involved in hearing, and diffusion impairment with regard to the formation of the lymph of the inner ear. DMSO would therefore appear to be an obvious choice as a basic treatment for tinnitus. DMSO expands the blood capillaries and can, as a 'taxi', improve diffusion processes in both directions. Depending on what the diagnosed cause is, it may also be advisable to administer other treatments. These may include taking oxidants (MMS, H_2O_2) if the tinnitus is caused by an inflammation, infection or autoimmune reaction, or undergoing hyperbaric oxygen therapy if the main cause is oxygen deficiency (e.g. in the case of smokers, or those suffering from lung diseases, cardiac insufficiency, etc.). From a holistic perspective, tinnitus is often regarded as being caused by too much stress and / or an imbalance in the internal physiological environment. It is therefore a symptom that should be taken very seriously. The first and most important measures that should be taken are rest and water ... plenty of water.

DMSO can be used locally or internally to treat tinnitus. Ideally, combine the two methods. For topical administration, use aqueous solutions of about 40 to 50% DMSO. Lie on one side, administer 2 to 3 drops into the ear canal and remain in that position for 20 minutes. Then, if necessary, repeat on the other side. Any of the three methods described in Chapter 2 can be used for internal application: moisten a large area of skin with a 70% DMSO solution, drink a heavily diluted solution (initial dose of 3.5ml DMSO in a 300ml drink), or infusions starting at 0.1g DMSO per kilogram of body weight.

Torn ligaments (see also Sports injuries)

Dr Morton Walker describes the following case in his book.[19] Retired teacher Gertie Brown, then 62 years old, had injured her knee in January 1980 and suffered terrible pain. At times she could not move. The orthopaedist diagnosed a torn ligament and told her that she would have to undergo an operation. She refused. Six months later she heard of the excellent results achieved using DMSO and she sought treatment at Dr William Campbell Douglass' clinic. She applied DMSO externally to the knee and was given eight infusions at relatively low doses. Gertie Brown began treating other joints that had become painful over the years. All her pains disappeared. The knee continued to feel weak and did not recover all its strength, which is only to be expected after suffering a torn ligament. Since then she has been applying a small dose of DMSO to the knee before going to bed each night and as a result is able to carry out her daily tasks. She is very satisfied and is happy to have avoided surgery.

Urinary tract infections

In the US, pure DMSO is only officially approved for use as a treatment for the non-bacterial form of bladder infection, known as interstitial cystitis. Experience has shown, however, that a number of 'normal' urinary tract infections can also be effectively treated using DMSO. Because of the dynamics of elimination following internal administration, DMSO quickly reaches the efferent urinary tract via the kidneys and can, as a result, easily reach any inflammation in both ureters, the bladder and the urethra. Doctors and alternative practitioners favour infusion as a method of administration.

In one of the many clinical trials conducted in the USA on DMSO as a treatment for urinary tract and bladder infections, 213 patients were treated using DMSO, all of whom had undergone other treatments without success. The condition of each and every patient improved, and their health problems disappeared without needing the operations that would otherwise have been necessary.

Varicose veins

This condition leads to parts of the surface veins of the legs becoming knotty and enlarged when sitting and standing due to the force the blood exerts on the weak walls of the veins. This process, which develops over a long period of time, is most commonly caused by a weakness of the tissue and is contingent on the individual's genetic makeup. There are, however, other causes of varicose veins, including a preceding thrombosis, tumours and injuries (from accidents) with scarring. The veins in the legs become enlarged and the valves which normally prevent the blood from flowing backwards are no longer able to close tightly. DMSO is clearly able to improve the tissue tonus, thereby improving the functionality of the vessel walls. This may be linked to an improved supply to the various layers of the walls in the large veins. Capillary expansion and improved diffusion could both be contributing factors. Together with applying the aqueous DMSO solution to the affected part of the leg or to the whole leg, infusions are highly recommended because the vessel and the venous system is then flooded with high concentrations of the active substance. After carrying out the tolerance test, start with 0.1 grams of DMSO per kilogram of body weight mixed in a 250 or 500ml infusion.

Case: male, 71 years old, had extensive varicose vein formations on the lower leg, accompanied by pressure pains. A keen experimenter, he brushed this area regularly with a 70% DMSO solution and was delighted to observe that the varicose veins were noticeably reduced after a few weeks. The pain disappeared, as did the feeling of heaviness in the legs.

Case: Ms K. F., 47 years old, suffers from enlarged varicose vein formations and venous thrombosis. Due to the chronic blood stasis, surface lesions (that are very difficult to cure) form mainly on the lower legs. Following my advice she has so far undergone two DMSO infusion treatments at the starting dose; she reported soon after that the stasis symptoms had significantly decreased. She is keen to continue with this treatment.

Withdrawal symptoms

Withdrawal symptoms arise as a result of reducing the dose or abstaining from a drug following an addiction. The most common addictions include alcohol, nicotine, tranquilizers (e.g. Valium® / diazepam) and opiates (e.g. heroin, morphine). The term 'drug' has a wide range of uses; in the scientific and pharmaceutical context it denotes (plant) medicinal substances generally. Historically, this word did not have negative connotations. It has only become the generally accepted term for potentially addictive substances because it originally referred to pure plant sub stances (e g. from opium poppy). This is not the place to discuss the vast range of different (political / legal) classifications of the abovementioned 'addictive substances'. It is, however, a fact that alcohol and nicotine, both of which are legal, have a much greater negative impact on the health of the nation than other drugs. I am of the opinion that we could easily extend the list of addictive and dangerous substances. What about the flavour enhancers and the other approved additives contained in much of today's (convenience) food? What about caffeine? Did evolution intend for us humans to need caffeine in order to get going every morning? Unpleasant and sometimes unbearable symptoms develop as a result of the daily consumption of what we may not usually consider to be drugs. Television, computer games, betting, information, sport and a certain relationship could all be included here. Regarding almost all addictive habits, the affected person usually exhibits very little if any awareness of his / her situation. You have probably heard smokers say: 'I could quit at any time!' This general lack of comprehension – a characteristic of addictive behaviour – accounts for the fact that change often comes too late, if at all.

Once the decision has been made to abstain from addictive and compulsive behaviours or substances, the person concerned will be faced with withdrawal symptoms that can last for varying periods of time. The symptoms, which can all arise simultaneously or consecutively, vary greatly. They include heart and circulation fluctuations, vegetative disturbances (e.g. sweating, tremors), hormone and metabolic dysfunctions, pain, as well as the much-feared subjective symptoms of anxiety, nervousness, aggression, and concentration and sleep problems. These symptoms indicate that addictions have an enormous influence on the chemical messenger balance in the central nervous system and on the circadian rhythm. Depending on the initial situation, withdrawal and weaning periods should be supervised by a professional, as should any subsequent period of resocialisation. DMSO is a helpful basic measure for the period of time during which doses of the addictive substance are reduced or discontinued. This is because it has a pain-relieving, detoxifying and regenerative effect. It can be taken as a drink or via infusion.

In some cases it may be advisable to apply it to large areas of the skin. The prickling and itching sensations caused by this substance can focus the patient's attention on the health-promoting measures being undertaken, and this can have an emotionally stabilising and reassuring effect. The withdrawal symptoms may then retreat into the background somewhat, and the patient's attention is directed towards healing.

The dose used for any of the three application methods should be set at or around the lower levels suggested in Chapter 2. Although DMSO accelerates the elimination of addictive substances, their metabolites and other toxins, it can also intensify the (remaining) effect of those substances. Even in cases of addictions not involving substances, the body should be given the time it needs to slowly correct the concentrations of neurotransmitters, hormones and metabolic products that have become out of balance. The whole process of working towards freedom from addiction should be accompanied by a holistic range of measures. These include measures to stabilise the acid–alkaline balance, stress-reduction measures and talking therapy. It really is worth it! Along with curing yourself of a chronic disease, you will be regaining a huge amount of personal freedom – as if you were winning your own very personal civil war.

Wounds

A wound is a type of injury where the outermost layer of skin is torn or punctured. Wounds can occur as a result of acute injuries, burns or accidents, or they can form over long periods of time, such as pressure sores (bedsores) or venous ulcers (ulcus cruris). The first priority is disinfection, whether the wound was caused by animal bites, bike accidents, injuries caused by tools, glass shards, burns / frostbites or ulcers. But you should avoid using the alcohol-based disinfectants that are common today. Instead, use good old hydrogen peroxide (about 1 to 3%) or calcium hypochlorite solution (about 1 teaspoon in ½-litre of water). Applied by spraying, these preparations are gentle on the skin that is still healthy, making it easier for the wound to heal. We can even expect these oxidative substances to activate the affected tissue in a very positive way. This is often reported in various internet discussion forums. Such statements also accord with the explanations given in Chapter 2.5 of this book regarding combinations of oxidative substances (MMS, H_2O_2) and DMSO. Immediately after the wound has been disinfected, DMSO can be sprayed over the wound and left to exert its healing effect.

DMSO, with its comprehensive regenerative effects, supports all repair processes. You will be amazed by the degree to which the 50 to 75% DMSO solutions used for this purpose improve the speed and quality of wound closure at every stage of recovery. It also minimises or completely prevents the wound from hardening and prevents adhesions from forming. In my opinion this substance's wonderful ability to heal is never so evident or so lovely to see as when treating (skin) injuries. Any inflammation in or damage to deeper-lying tissue is also treated. It is important to allow the wound to be in contact with air as much as possible. The common mistake of applying plasters to the smallest of cuts only leads to exuding wounds and avoidable inflammation or infection. Once you have disinfected the wound it is best to leave the area to dry. Moreover, the itching and skin redness caused by DMSO is less pronounced if the wound is left uncovered.

Case: Mr R. M., 64 years old, diabetic, suffered an accident about a year ago in which a palette fell on his foot. The wound along the side of his big toe had never healed and he suffered permanent and severe pain. This pain, which had caused him so much suffering for such a long time, abated after two spray applications of a 75% DMSO solution. After a further week of DMSO treatment (two applications a day) a scab formed and the wound healed completely.

Case: Mr M. G., 45 years old, had been suffering from a 20cm-long venous ulcer for a long time, presumably because of venous insufficiency. On my suggestion he took an MMS leg bath once, and subsequently applied a 75% DMSO solution to the affected area every day for a month. The wound healed without complications and full muscle function was restored.

Case: A. G., 5 years old, had jammed the fingers of his left hand in the door while getting out of the car. The fingertips and nails were badly injured and he cried constantly because of the pain. With incredible presence of mind, his father reached for a bottle of DMSO, which he had to hand because of another illness, and sprayed this 80% solution over his son's hand. After a few minutes the pain subsided. Further treatment brought about swift healing and the fingers were back to normal within a few days.

Case: Ms A. F., 51 years old, had undergone an ankle operation six months previously after suffering a splintered fracture. Although the operation went well, the surgical wound would not heal. This resulted in necrosis of the tissue and a *Staphylococcus* infection (pyogenic bacteria). After suffering for so long, Ms F. followed my advice and took an MMS bath then treated the wound with a 75% DMSO solution every day. The inflammation disappeared and the wound healed completely within two weeks.

Morton Walker[19] cites 1,371(!) cases in which patients experienced unambiguously positive results following topical DMSO treatment. These patients suffered from ulcers on the legs, feet and hips as a result of diabetes, fungal infections or varicose veins, infected wounds, various forms of damaged skin, and second and third degree burns. After washing the skin using only sterile water, they were treated using DMSO sprays daily at first, and then three times a week. In most cases, the pain and discomfort abated after just a few applications. After 20 days, 95% of those treated were discharged and deemed to be totally cured and were able to resume their usual activities, even though some of them had suffered the ulcers for many years.[71] Chronic inflammatory varicose vein ulcers that had been treated in the conventional manner for many years without success, also quickly healed. Burns on the arms healed without scarring of any kind. Dr Rene Miranda Tirado, the leading doctor on the study, is quoted as saying, 'The DMSO spray did the job.' The only side effect mentioned is that the spray causes a burning sensation of varying severity for a short while after it is used for the first few times on very deep wounds. In all these cases, this highly effective DMSO treatment was continued in response to requests by patients.

DMSO FOR ANIMALS

In theory, all the information given in the preceding chapters regarding DMSO doses, fields of application and methods of use, are also valid when using DMSO to treat other mammals. However, there are obvious differences that must be taken into consideration, such as physical structure, lack of comprehension of the treatment, and a compulsion to move.

Firstly, higher doses of DMSO can usually be given to animals. This is because certain losses must be allowed for (or at least when we are not dealing with infusions). An animal might not drink the DMSO solution in its entirety, or it may partially rub off DMSO solutions that are applied externally. External application is particularly problematic in the case of dogs, cats, etc. because of the coat. If the affected area is covered by thick fur and you do not want to (or cannot) shave that area, you can apply a higher dose just to be on the safe side. Make certain that the DMSO reaches the animal's skin. Stiff brushes can be used to massage the liquid into the skin. DMSO preparations that adhere to the body can be prepared by mixing DMSO with aloe vera gel instead of with water. The ratio is the same as when using water, e.g. 70ml DMSO plus 30ml aloe vera gel.

External application is used mainly to treat diseases of the musculoskeletal system, particularly the limbs. You can use DMSO on your own initiative to treat inflamed joints, injuries, swelling, and symptoms of overexertion suffered by pets, sporting animals and working animals. The same concentrations of DMSO can be used on animals as were listed in Chapter 2 for use on humans. For example, dilutions of about 60 to 75% can be used externally on the limbs. Ear, nose and eye drops are also included in the category 'external applications' (always use sterile solutions).

High concentrations of aqueous DMSO solutions can be used to rinse out wounds, ulcers, abscesses or fistulas. To do so, use a plastic dropper bottle or plastic syringe and apply the 50 to 80% solution directly to the affected area.

There is a number of officially approved medications containing

DMSO that can be used to treat animals externally / topically (see Chapter 2.1); a vet will be able to prescribe these for you. However, these are all mixtures of DMSO and other medications such as cortisone or antibiotics. They are available as creams, gels and drops, but most of these products only contain small quantities of DMSO.

DMSO can be used internally on animals suffering from muscle, joint and bone conditions. All the human diseases listed in Chapter 3 can be treated in the same way in the case of animals. You will need to be creative because you cannot expect an animal to understand or intuit why it should drink a liquid that has an unusual taste, and you will certainly not be able to expect it to drink all the liquid, and that in separate doses divided over the course of a day. To give you an example: there was a Viennese rabbit that was to be treated using DMSO because it suffered from extensive eczema. It would not touch the water in its bottle initially so its owners did not give it any fresh green food for a little while, as they would normally have done at that time of year, only some dry pellets. The rabbit soon became thirsty after eating and it was 'forced' to drink from the bottle since it had no other alternative. This shows how you can direct DMSO treatment when the animal is living within a confined space.

Treating 'free spirits' such as dogs, horses and, above all, cats is quite a different proposition. These animals are usually (one would hope) free to roam outside and they do not like to be dictated to. In these cases you have to either administer the drink solution during the time the animal spends indoors or try your luck adjusting the taste by mixing DMSO with a variety of different drinks. Perhaps you need to exercise a little patience while the animal becomes accustomed to the new taste / smell. I am told that some animals are happy to drink DMSO immediately … possibly because they intuitively sense its healing effect. In the case of other small animals it is possible to administer DMSO directly into the mouth using a pipette.

The dose for internal use is based roughly on the animal's weight although, as mentioned above, you do not need to be afraid of being a little generous. If a dog weighing 15kg is to be given DMSO treatment at a dose of 0.5g per kg of body weight, a dose of 7.5g of pure DMSO, or about 7ml would be required. But bearing in mind that this quantity is put into the dog's water bowl and that some of this might be spilled or left behind in the bowl, you can give 10ml without worry. That is roughly equivalent to three teaspoons.

Infusions are a good means of ensuring that a specific quantity of DMSO is given to an animal, but they are usually difficult to administer at home. This method of treatment is widely used in equestrian sport, where DMSO infusions are used to treat all manner of joint problems. DMSO infusions are also used on performance horses as a regenerative substance following operations and injuries. A well-known horse healer in northern Germany was featured in a television documentary 'prescribing' this method of treatment for a sports horse.

Standard doses are about 300 grams(!) of DMSO in a 2.5 litre infusion. If you believe DMSO could help your animals, you can ask your vet about the possibility of administering such a treatment. Many of you might be a little hesitant initially because DMSO has not been officially approved as a medication[*] for animals and because you are not allowed to use it on farm animals (pigs, dairy cows, etc.) for bureaucratic reasons. Animals that produce meat, milk or any other products are subject to the most stringent controls. Vets and farmers are only allowed to use approved medications, which must all be documented in detail, when treating such animals – that is comparable to a planned economy. But it is not so in the case of animals that are kept as pets or for sport. The owner is free to decide how their animals are treated or fed.

Anyone who knows or lives in the vicinity of Karin Fietzner, an alternative health practitioner, is very lucky indeed. She is just as happy treating humans as she is treating animals, and she has extensive experience in this field. Her practice is based in Linden, Germany, and she has a farm in nearby Romrod, where she can accommodate a limited number of animals, large and small, that have been tortured, mistreated or 'winnowed' for whatever reason (www.naturheilpraxis-fietzner.de). At the moment she is treating her mare, Riccina, for laminitis using DMSO, CDS (chlorine dioxide solution) and superoxide infusions, by following an appropriate staggered timetable that I suggested.

The images below show how Riccina is treated using a DMSO infusion. It is clear from figure 42 that the sick horse usually tries to spare the afflicted front hooves by moving some of the weight onto the back hooves. After the infusion has been flowing for a few minutes (figure 43) she becomes more relaxed and spreads her weight evenly over four legs. I also recommended MMS and / or H_2O_2 foot baths.

---

[*] News: As of November 2015 DMSO ampules are officially available in Germany!

During the course of this treatment we noticed something that supports a theory I have been developing. Riccina was given a medium dose of DMSO by infusion and soon exuded the infamous garlic odour to such an extent that even the neighbours noticed. Over the course of the treatment programme, and after using CDS, this odour became much less noticeable. That is why I believe that the reductive transformation of DMSO into gaseous dimethyl sulphide is less pronounced as the toxic load of the body is progressively reduced. In other words, the odour is stronger when the body is lacking in oxidative power (whether that is due to illness or toxic load), i.e. when the immune system is weakened. Since we are not usually able to observe human patients as closely because they leave the clinic after a treatment, or because they administer the treatment at home themselves, it had not been possible for me to confirm this hypothesis. If the intensity of the odour, i.e. the quantity of dimethyl sulphide produced in the body, really varies in line with the severity of the dysfunction, we could use this as an indicator of the patient's progress. In short, a weakened or toxic body produces more odour as a result of reductive metabolic processes than a healthy body, in which DMSO is almost completely oxidised into dimethyl sulfone (MSM) – a highly desirable effect. That, at least, is the theory. If you

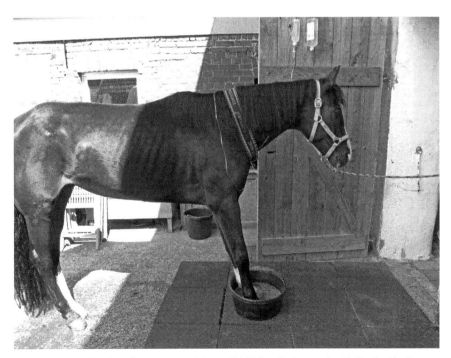

Figure 42: Riccina the mare receiving a DMSO infusion and a H_2O_2 footbath

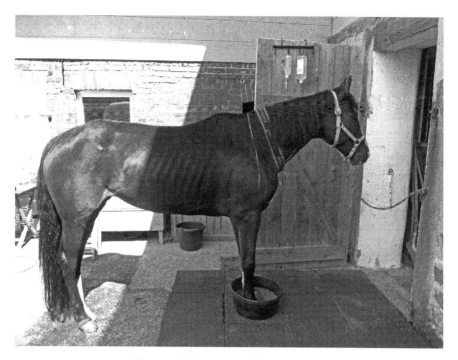

Figure 43: Riccina can relax once again

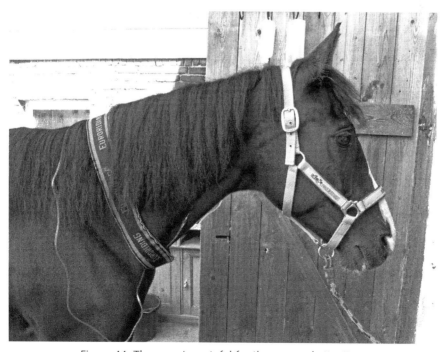

Figure 44: The mare is grateful for the care and attention

have experiences or observations in this regard, we would be very grateful if you could send them to us or to the publisher. Real-life experiences are often far more useful in terms of increasing and sharing knowledge than the more 'sterile' research carried out in laboratories, particularly considering that that avenue is closed as far as DMSO is concerned.

The intensity of the odour is, of course, first and foremost dependent on the individual's constitution and has to do with their metabolic state, especially the liver enzyme activity. As you know, different people can handle varying amounts of alcohol. Despite that, it appears that there is a significant reduction in the amount of dimethyl sulphide produced after the first treatment if the body becomes increasingly healthy. In the same way, I often notice that skin reactions to external applications (red skin, itching, etc.) are much subtler during subsequent treatments than they are as the result of the first application.

Karin Fietzner is an exceptionally gifted chiropractor and uses this method just as successfully to treat both humans and animals. As a result, she is known locally as the 'horse adjuster' or 'horse healer'.

Everything that was said in the previous chapters regarding possible combinations of DMSO and other (alternative) medical substances is just as true of their use on animals. For example, MMS or hydrogen peroxide (oxidative anti-infection substances) can be mixed into the drinking-water at any time, in alternation with DMSO. Dr Tucker's cancer treatment, which uses a mixture of DMSO and the natural substance haematoxylin, has been shown to be very effective for treating dogs.[16] Animals that are well exercised, or working animals can, in my opinion, be given preventative DMSO treatment. Susceptibility to injury and illness is reduced and they enjoy increased energy because DMSO and its main metabolite MSM ensure a plentiful supply of organic sulphur to the body tissue. This also makes the joints and the musculature strong and flexible.

Until now I have only mentioned mammals. We can assume that a number of physiological processes, including the metabolic processing of DMSO, are either the same in mammals as they are in humans, or are similar. Scientifically speaking this is, of course, a serious oversimplification but it suffices for the purposes of this discussion. Excretion and tissue reactions such as inflammations proceed slightly differently in animals. An example of this is the superior internal repair function that other mammals have to heal wounds, whereby allantoin is produced from the metabolic product uric acid. Hominids cannot produce this because we lack the respective enzyme; uric acid is excreted 'unused', or can even be the cause of gout if too much is present in the blood. However, allantoin is available to humans if we eat foods containing the substance (black salsify, green beans, cauliflower, etc.) or in the form of a cosmetic additive for the treatment of skin. To return to DMSO use in animals, however, with regard to birds, reptiles, fish and insects, we only have individual experience reports by people who, at one time or another, hit upon the idea of dipping into their DMSO supplies for the benefit of their exotic household pets. It would be great if readers contacted us with descriptions of DMSO treatments given to such animals so that we can expand our database of cases. For example, DMSO could be added to the water in fish tanks or terrariums, possibly alternating it with MMS. Adding DMSO to drinking-water given to birds also appears to be a good idea.

It is conceivable that one could treat a bee colony by placing a shallow bowl on the base of the hive. Parasites have long developed resistance to the synthetic substances officially approved in order to combat mite infestations (*Varroa destructor*). Formic acid, oxalic acid and lactic acid, the natural substances used against *Varroa* mites, are often unsafe, or are not effective enough. Combining DMSO and MMS could be a new, easy-to-use alternative treatment for bee populations. There have already been initial successes in this regard.

SOURCES OF SUPPLY

U nfortunately we cannot name here those retailers whom we regard as being reliable suppliers of good quality products at reasonable prices. We refrain from naming them in order to avoid causing problems for them. In the past, recommendations made in public regarding reliable sources of certain substances resulted in pressures of various kinds being placed on those companies by the authorities and by representatives of certain interests. To continue to make public recommendations would be to saw off the branch we are sitting on as there is a danger that it could become increasingly difficult to obtain DMSO & Co. If you feel the advice provided here is not sufficient to guide you to a suitable retailer, contact the publisher. You might also want to consider expanding your knowledge of this field at one of our workshops (www.PraNatu.de).

Alpha lipoic acid

A number of companies sell alpha lipoic acid in the form of 600mg capsules or tablets. It is also available under different brand names in 50ml vials or infusion bottles. It is worth comparing prices. Buy from pharmacies. One gram of alpha lipoic acid in tablet form costs from about 40 pence.

Ascorbic acid

Also known as vitamin C, this substance can be bought in three different forms. Firstly, it is available as a pure, colourless powder for human consumption in package sizes of 50g, 100g or more, and can be found in health food shops, supermarkets and pharmacies. Secondly, it is available in ready-to-use tablets, capsules and effervescent tablets etc., usually containing between 100 and 1000 milligrams of ascorbic acid. These are also available in pharmacies and large stores. Thirdly, it is available as sterile, aqueous solutions in pharmaceutical vials (e.g. 500, 750 or 1000mg) or injection bottles (e.g. 7.5g in 50 millilitres) for intravenous administration. These are also available to buy over the counter and are produced by companies such as Pascoe, Dr Loges and Wörwag. There are sometimes significant price differences. High doses must be diluted in an isotonic infusion solution before intravenous use.

It should be noted that it is generally more difficult to absorb the free ascorbic acid in / from an acidic solution (such as an effervescent tablet). It is much more easily absorbed when the ascorbate is in an alkaline solution.

Calcium hypochlorite

Calcium hypochlorite, or $Ca(OCl)_2$, is the base substance used in MMS 2. It is available from chemical and swimming pool suppliers in the form of a 70% (approx.) white powder. Sales to private persons are restricted because it is classed as a dangerous substance due to its tendency to self-decompose. Prices range from £15 to £25 per kilogram. It must be stored in a dry place and as far away from other materials as possible. To use it as an aqueous solution to disinfect wounds, or as a bath additive, etc., pour and stir the required quantity of the calcium hypochlorite powder into a certain volume of water measured beforehand.

DMSO

These days, pure or pharmaceutical quality (min. 99.8%) DMSO is available from a number of internet retailers, chemical suppliers and pharmacies. But be aware that some retailers are still selling poor quality and / or overpriced products. DMSO should be completely odourless and colourless and there should be no liquid residue when it becomes solid at temperatures of below 18.5 °C. One kilogram of DMSO which meets European Pharmacopoeia standards (Ph. Eur.) usually costs between £25 and £35. Smaller quantities of about 100ml naturally cost more in proportion.

Every now and again I hear stories of how little pharmacists and country doctors know about the documented properties of DMSO. People in these professions often resort to scare tactics and a paradoxical overreaction, apparently because they feel the need to protect the source of their income and the position of power they derive from their medical authority. These 'knowledgeable' people unnerve their customers and patients by telling them that DMSO is 'banned' or 'poisonous'. But we should make one thing clear: **DMSO is a legally available substance and is an ingredient in a number of medications for humans and animals throughout the world.** Countless medical, physiological and pharmacological safety studies have shown that it is practically impossible to reach a toxic threshold because the quantities necessary are so high that It is inconceivable that a human could ingest so much. DMSO is far safer than most common medications, and other natural substances such as caffeine and cooking salt.

Effective microorganisms (EM)

These are available as pure culture solutions or as ready-to-use liquids containing prebiotic additives, which can include lactic acid bacteria, yeast and photosynthetic bacteria. While officially only recognised as a 'soil enhancer', their general and therapeutic uses and effects are just as varied as they are astonishing. They can be used as a quick solution to many skin problems, as an aid to regulate the intestinal flora, or as a natural way to improve the quality of air in a room. These cultures are sure to satisfy. They can be easily found on the internet by searching for 'effective microorganisms'. With a little skill and the appropriate nutrient solutions, you can even cultivate EM yourself. This is highly recommended because the ready-to-use products are very expensive.

Galactose

Galactose is available as a white powder and resembles glucose in appearance. However, it is much more expensive than glucose because the production process is quite complex and the quantities produced are much smaller. It really is worth searching for a cheap retailer / pharmacy on the internet as 500 grams can cost between £70 and £110.

Haematoxylin

This is a beige-coloured natural substance in powder form. It is mainly used as a dye in microscopy in the fields of biology, physiology and pathology. When dealing with laboratory suppliers, make certain that you are acquiring the pure substance. This is because you are often presented with ready-to-use liquid preparations containing additional ingredients that are normally used to prepare samples in microscope analysis. Normally, 100 grams of the pure powder costs about £160.

Hydrogen peroxide

This substance can be purchased in various concentrations in pharmacies or from chemical suppliers. Pharmacies in Germany usually stock 1.5 to 3% H_2O_2 preparations that are certified by the German Pharmacopeia (labelled as 'Hydrogen peroxide 3% DAB 11'). A litre costs between £2 and £6 and it can be used as it is without further preparation.

If you want to prepare other concentrations yourself, it is recommended that you buy a 30% Ph. Eur. grade hydrogen peroxide solution. Caution: it is highly corrosive! This can be diluted with the appropriate volume of water (use safety glasses and suitable gloves). Retailers usually require a 'proof of use', an 'end-user declaration' or a 'certificate of competence' for those higher concentrations. This is because they are classed as dangerous substances and because fanatical murderers use it to produce a certain kind of liquid explosive every now and then. This is a classic example of how the same substance can be used both to help and to harm humanity. We are all clearly connected by a single global consciousness and we should turn towards our fellow man with benevolence, not with murderous hate.

Low concentrations of hydrogen peroxide have a surprising number of uses and benefits – it really is worth learning what those are, and experimenting.

Infusion solutions

You can obtain infusion solutions complete with all the accessories in a range of varieties at (online) pharmacies. For the kind of applications described in this book we normally use infusion bottles (glass or plastic) containing 500 or 1000ml of sterile, isotonic saline solution (= 0.9% NaCl solution). The main difference between the most common varieties (Braun, Fresenius, etc.) is the quality of the pierceable membrane. Some of these are so tight or 'stubborn' that it can be very difficult to push through the infusion set or to inject substances into them. The volumes they contain can also vary greatly. There are infusion bottles that are not completely filled with the isotonic base substance so that large quantities of other liquid substances can be added. Experiment and learn as you go. We cover all the options and price variations in our workshops and seminars. You can also learn how to produce and self-administer various infusion solutions.

(+) – lactic acid

Right-turning lactic acid is widely available as a 21% solution from pharmacies and internet health food shops. In this form it can be added to drinks or used as an activator for MMS. Higher concentrations of right-turning lactic acid can be bought from chemical suppliers. By diluting these with appropriate quantities of purified water, you can prepare ready-to-use solutions of about 20%.

MMS / CDS

MMS and CDS can be bought from a number of internet retailers and the prices are generally similar (e.g. MMS Lotus 2 x 100ml for about £20). The original MMS is usually sold in sets of two bottles, i.e. the 22.4% aqueous sodium chlorite solution and the activator. The activator is usually an appropriate concentration of citric, tartaric or hydrochloric acid. If you intend to use a different activator (e.g. lactic acid, sodium bisulfate, vinegar) you will need to search for stockists who sell sodium chlorite solution separately. Another very affordable option is to buy pure sodium chlorite in powder form (from chemical or swimming pool suppliers) and produce the 22.4% aqueous solution yourself. Some wholesalers now offer the 22.4% solution. The only drawback is that pure sodium chlorite is classed as a dangerous substance due to its corrosive effects and it cannot officially be sold to everyone and anyone. Moreover, as a private user you usually only need small quantities, certainly not barrel-loads, unless you intend to take regular MMS baths or disinfect your private swimming pool with it. It is worth repeating that sodium chlorite and chlorine dioxide (the substance that is produced through activation) are approved under the German Drinking Water Ordinance and are used in rich countries (and households) to purify bathing water. In contrast to chlorine, which is known to be harmful to health, chlorine dioxide solutions in the recommended concentrations have extremely positive effects on health. It is, therefore, misleading to claim that MMS / sodium chlorite use 'on humans' is banned. We can and should understand the threats coming from various authorities and hidden 'backers' as being motivated by the selfish interests of the pharmaceutical industry. When we consider the current legal situation and the extensive data on the safety of $NaClO_2$, we can relax. Not only is this substance widely used to purify drinking- and bathing water, it has also been used in the food industry and in other sectors for a long time to treat water and to kill microorganisms. We can happily accept that retailers are not allowed to label it as a health treatment; we simply put that down to the typical bureaucracy of our time, and continue doing what we are already doing in order to support good health.

The newer chlorine dioxide solutions (CDS) contain the active substance MMS – gaseous chlorine dioxide (ClO_2) – in its pure form. Chlorine dioxide solutions are ready-to-use solutions and do not require activation. As a rule, these are labelled as <0.29% solutions because that means that they are not classed as dangerous substances and that they can be sent by standard post. Bottles should be stored in a cool, dark place and should always be closed tightly. At room temperature, chlorine dioxide can quickly escape and it breaks down when exposed to light or impurities. However, CDS in unopened violet bottles can be stored for more than a year with only minimal loss of content. Learn how to produce fresh chlorine dioxide solutions in appropriate concentrations using simple techniques at my workshops.

Procaine

Procaine is available over the counter in 2 and 5ml vials as a 0.5 to 2.0% solution in the form of procaine hydrochloride. Well-known manufacturers include Pascoe, Loges, Hevert, Steigerwald, etc. Depending on the quantity you buy, a 2ml vial of a 1% procaine solution costs between 25 pence and £1. It is therefore worth comparing prices. Procaine solutions can be injected as they are, or combined with other substances (sodium bicarbonate, DMSO, homeopathic remedies, etc.). Health practitioners often have their own favourite combinations for treating various illnesses. Intracutaneous injections, clearing scar interference fields using the Hunecke method, and 'substance-based acupuncture' are only a few of the application possibilities of this tried-and-tested medication.

Purified water

You can either buy purified water or prepare your own. We make a distinction between salt-free and salt-containing water, and between sterile and non-sterile water. Salt-free water is usually labelled as 'distilled water' and is often sold in 5-litre bottles for the purpose of refilling car batteries and steam irons. As a rule it is not in actual fact distilled, but is either ultrafiltrated or has undergone a process known as reverse osmosis (RO-water). A range of different reverse osmosis equipment is now available for home use so that you can prepare salt-free, non-sterile water at any time. The RO filter membrane not only removes common salt ions such as sodium, calcium, sulphate, etc., from normal drinking-water, it also removes microorganisms, heavy metals, sedimentary elements and medication residues. These appliances are available as standard equipment for kitchens – some of them have their own in-built containers while others allow the water to run into a glass jug placed at a lower level. Some are connected to the main water supply while others are filled by hand. There is a large choice of appliances, and reverse osmosis water is suitable for all uses Whether you want to use it to prepare tea, soak whole grains or prepare medications, you will notice a difference when you use purified water. Distilled water, i.e. water prepared by vaporisation and condensation, is available from chemical suppliers and pharmacies. It is completely free of salt but is not sterile.

If you require purified but not salt-free water, remineralise the RO or distilled water with a full-spectrum sea or rock salt. Use your intuition and add a pinch to the water. However, if you are preparing isotonic water, you need to calculate the quantity of salt more precisely. Isotonic water has an electrolyte content of 0.9%, which means that 9 grams of salt is dissolved in one litre of water. Purified and remineralised water is perfect for diluting DMSO solutions, whether for external application or to be taken as a drink.

Sterile, isotonic water must always be used when preparing dilutions that are to be used as ear, eye or nose drops, and even more importantly for infusion solutions!

How or where can you source this type of water? Very simply: buy ready-to-use infusion solutions in glass or plastic bottles / bags in the desired size and quantity from an (online) pharmacy. It should state 'sterile isotonic saline solution' or 'sterile 0.9% NaCl solution' on the label. These infusion solutions are available over the counter in sizes of between 100ml and 1 litre at very affordable prices. To prepare DMSO dilutions that will not be administered by infusion, the required quantity of this sterile water is extracted from the bottle or bag via the pierceable membrane using a cannula (yellow) and a syringe. When preparing infusion solutions, follow the instructions given in Chapter 2.4.

Summary: distilled water – i.e. purified, salt-free water – can be bought in pharmacies, chemists and supermarkets, or it can be produced at home using reverse osmosis equipment. The water can be remineralised by adding up to 9 grams of full-spectrum natural salt per litre (isotonic). This kind of water is not sterile.

If you require sterile water, for example when preparing ear drops, when treating open wounds, or for injections / infusions, you can buy sterile, isotonic infusion liquids in bottles or bags at your local pharmacy. These are 0.9% sodium chloride solutions.

Sodium bicarbonate

Also known as baking soda and bicarbonate of soda. Its chemical formula is $NaHCO_3$. Sodium bicarbonate for medical use is available in two main forms that are of interest to us. Firstly, it can be bought as a white powder in a variety of purity grades. Secondly, it is available as a sterile 8.4% infusion and injection solution to alkalise doses of medication that are to be administered using these two methods.

Pure sodium bicarbonate in powder form has a wide range of uses. It is an ingredient used in baking powder, (effervescent) tablets and soda water. It is a tried-and-tested remedy for heartburn. When the topic of sodium bicarbonate came up Professor Max Schmidt, the 'cult professor' who moulded the introductory chemistry lecture course for all science and medicine students at the University of Würzburg in the 1980s and early 1990s, always used to refer to the old advertising slogan: 'Just as you need a bride at a wedding, you need Bullrich Salts to help with digesting.' Bullrich Salts contains 100% sodium bicarbonate and has none of the side effects of PPIs. It is also used in bath additives, toothpastes, cleaning products, and it is used in industry as a water softener and a food additive (acidity regulator E500). It is used as an agricultural antifungal agent, to stabilise pH values in pools and aquariums, and to 'cut' illegal drugs. In short, you can acquire good quality, cheap sodium bicarbonate in powder form anywhere (e.g. supermarkets, health food shops, pharmacies). We use it as an acidity regulator in a number of preparations.

You can only buy the sterile 8.4% ready-to-use solutions in pharmacies. These are used as alkaline infusions (see Chapter 2.5.2) to treat acidosis or are used in combination with procaine to increase its effect. A 250ml bottle costs at least £5 to £7 pounds assuming the retailer uses scaled pricing. The required quantities can be taken from the bottle using a syringe cannula or a spike (with a valve and a Luer lock) that can be left in the bottle septum for multiple use.

Other useful equipment

You will need equipment for measuring, handling and using DMSO and other substances if you wish to move beyond the basic applications and uses. Graduated pipettes and cylinders, syringes, cannulas and filters are usually available for a few pennies. For example, when bought in packets of 100, a cannula costs a penny or two, a 10ml syringe costs about 5 pence, and an injection filter (pore size 200 nanometer) costs about £1 to £2. You can acquire these from pharmacies, wholesalers, medical suppliers or you can 'go begging' for them from any doctors or health practitioners you may know. The same is true for other equipment such as swabs, single-use gloves, infusion sets, 'butterflies' or winged infusion sets, disinfection sprays, tourniquets, etc. Having said that, I should emphasise once again that you can achieve amazing results using only the most basic equipment such as brushes, teaspoons, egg cups, etc. Do not be afraid of getting started; make the most of these wonderful, cost-efficient possibilities.

OVERVIEW OF DOSES

B elow you will find a summary of DMSO application methods and doses. Even though DMSO is extremely well tolerated and has a very high LD_{50} value, you should always start with low doses when administering self-treatment.

Quantity indications always refer to pure DMSO (Ph. Eur., produced in accordance with European Pharmacopoeia regulations) at concentrations of about 99.8%. Always check the label because a number of internet retailers also offer pre-mixed 70% solutions or less.

For practical tips on measuring, mixing and storing DMSO, see Chapter 2. For information on what type of water to use, see Chapter 5.

Always carry out a tolerance test before using DMSO for the first time (see Chapter 2.2).

EXTERNAL APPLICATION TO THE SKIN

Never use pure DMSO! Always prepare a diluted solution at appropriate concentrations. For example, to prepare a 60% DMSO solution, mix 6 parts of pure DMSO with 4 parts water.

Appropriate concentrations for external applications:

Feet / legs: 60–80% aqueous DMSO solution
Torso / arms: 40–70% aqueous DMSO solution
Neck / head: 35–50% aqueous DMSO solution
Ear / nose drops: 25–50% isotonic, aqueous DMSO solution
Open wounds: 30–60% sterile, isotonic, aqueous DMSO solution
Skin warts: 80–90% aqueous solution, dabbed onto skin using cotton swabs
Eye drops
(special application):   0.5% sterile, isotonic, aqueous DMSO solution

DMSO is usually administered once or twice a day. Because DMSO solutions are highly fluid, a few millilitres is usually enough to sufficiently moisten the skin. Because of this we usually pour a certain amount of the liquid into a glass; then use a brush, your hands, a cotton swab or a pipette to apply the liquid from this glass. You can buy sterile, isotonic water (for treating open wounds or to prepare eye drops) as infusion solutions in glass or plastic bottles in sizes ranging from 0.1 to 1 litre in any pharmacy.

If you wish to use DMSO in baths, the dose depends on what exactly you want to achieve. A few millilitres of DMSO is sufficient to improve the absorption of other substances in the bathwater (chloride dioxide or hydrogen peroxide, for example). Using larger quantities you will be able to feel the whole spectrum of DMSO's beneficial effects. However, the most effective way of absorbing DMSO, and to treat the skin using DMSO, is to administer it directly to the skin.

INTERNAL USE

Drinking highly diluted DMSO solutions is the easiest way of taking the substance. However, this method can, apparently, cause headaches, liver pain and dizziness at first. To supply the body with the desired quantity of DMSO it is sufficient to drink the mixture once a day, for example after breakfast.

The daily dose, i.e. the total quantity of DMSO administered daily in clinical trials, is calculated based on the patient's body weight. Standard doses are about 0.05–1 gram of DMSO per kilogram of body weight. For a person weighing 70kg, the dose administered would be between 3.5 and 70 grams or 3 to 65ml. **Pure DMSO should never be employed for internal use.** Always use highly diluted mixtures, using a maximum of 15ml (approx. 16.5g) of pure DMSO in a large glass containing 0.3 litres of water, juice or tea. Use a metal teaspoon as a simple measurement guide: 1 teaspoon is equal to about 3.5 grams of DMSO. **Add a maximum of 4 to 5 teaspoons of DMSO to a glass containing 0.3 litres of water, juice or tea.** If you want to take a higher daily dose, you will need to divide the dose between more than one drink.

DOSAGE EXAMPLES

Body weight	Starting dose	Maxium dose
40kg	2g	40g
50kg	2.5g	50g
60kg	3g	60g
70kg	3.5g	70g
80kg	4g	80g
90kg	4.5g	90g
100kg	5g	100g

For a mouthwash 5–20% aqueous solutions can be used. For example, you can mix 10 grams of pure DMSO (about 3 teaspoons) in 100ml of water, giving you a 10% solution. Specific areas of the oral mucosa affected by inflammation or injury can be dabbed with stronger concentrations of DMSO (up to 80%) using a cotton swab.

SEMINARS AND LECTURES

Hartmut Fischer, the author of this book, lectures and holds workshops on DMSO, MMS, CDS and other alternative medicines throughout Germany, Austria and Switzerland. For more details see the 'Seminars' page on www.PraNatu.de

AFTERWORD

In the process of reading this book you will have gained much knowledge about DMSO and the wonderful effects it can have on your health. Like me, you may have enjoyed this informative, lucid and clearly-written book so much, you may almost regret that it is coming to an end. The author imparts his knowledge in an extremely engaging manner and I am happy to admit that I have learned much despite being already familiar with the topic.

I am very pleased that Hartmut Fischer accepted the task of writing this book because without doubt he is more qualified to do so than anyone else I know (including myself). He has successfully integrated the knowledge he has gathered from his study of chemistry, from his pharmaceutical research, and from his practical experience of treating patients as an alternative health practitioner, and distilled it all into this book on DMSO. The result is this expert work that succeeds in explaining complex processes in a simple and comprehensible manner, drawing on years of experience to focus on only the most important aspects. In addition, Hartmut Fischer has included in this book a number of his own 'discoveries' and personal suggestions.

He was educated at a Gymnasium (grammar school) that took a humanistic approach, before moving on to study natural sciences in the Department of Chemistry and Pharmacology at the Julius Maximilian University of Würzburg in Bavaria. He then spent a number of years as a research scientist for major pharmaceutical companies. He worked on a German Research Foundation project, developing chiral syntheses, at the Institute for Organic Chemistry at the University of Würzburg, and spent a number of years working on development and application methods in water preparation. He took parental leave when both his children were born and felt compelled to follow a calling to become an alternative health practitioner. Along the way he also volunteered for the emergency medical service in the adult education department of the Bavarian Red Cross, and he trained as a hospice carer in Fulda.

His patients benefit enormously from his wealth of knowledge and experience, and he passes on his expertise by teaching on training courses for prospective alternative health practitioners and courses on DMSO and MMS use. You will find more details on his website www.PraNatu.de.

Hartmut Fischer combines profound scientific insights with a way of life that incorporates wisdom, compassion and inquisitiveness. Everything he says or writes testifies to his knowledge, his profundity, and the respect he shows towards his fellow men. What I most admire about him is his personal integrity. You can rest assured that everything written here was written with your highest good in mind. Hartmut Fischer has done what he could – and that achievement is invaluable. But now it is up to you to take full advantage of that. I wish you all the best!

With very best wishes,
Dr Antje Oswald

LIST OF REFERENCES

1 Muir, M., 'DMSO: Many Uses. Much Controversy', *Alternative and Complementary Therapies,* July/August 1996, 230–5

2 Kleberger, E., 'Linse mit doppeltem Brennpunkt (Butzenscheibenlinse) erzeugt durch toxische Dosen von Dimethylsulfoxyd (DMSO) an Hunden', *Graefe's Archive for Clinical and Experimental Ophthalmology,* 1967/173(3), 269–81

3 Wood, D. C., Wirth, N. V., 'Weitere Untersuchungen zur Wirkung von Dimethylsulfoxyd am Kaninchenauge', *DMSO-Symposium, Vienna,* Berlin / Saladruck, 1966, 58

4 Saytzeff [Zaitsev], A. M., 'Über die Einwirkung von Salpetersäure auf Schwefelmethyl und Schwefeläthyl', *Liebigs Annalen der Chemie und Pharmazie,* 1867, 144–8

5 Ueltschi, G., Schlatter, C., 'Effect of dimethyl sulfoxide on the percutaneous penetration of phenylbutazone and 3H-flumethasone', *Archiv für Experimentelle Veterinärmedizin,* 1974/28(1), 101–11

6 Layman, D. L., Jacob, S. W., 'The absorption, metabolism and excretion of dimethyl sulfoxide by rhesus monkeys', *Life Sciences,* 1985/37(25), 2431–7

7 Hucker, H. B., Miller, J. K., Hochberg, A., Brobyn, R. D., Riordan, F. H., Calesnick, B., 'Studies on the absorption, excretion and metabolism of dimethylsulfoxide (DMSO) in man', *The Journal of Pharmacology and Experimental Therapeutics,* 1967/155(2), 309–17

8 Gerhards, E., Gibian, H., 'Stoffwechsel und Wirkung des Dimethylsulfoxids', *Naturwissenschaften,* 1968/55(9), 435–8

9 Williams, K. I. H., Burstein, S. H., Layne, D. S., 'Dimethyl sulfone: Isolation from human urine', *Archives of Biochemistry and Biophysics,* 1966/113(1), 251–2

10 Kolb, K. H., Jaenicke, G., Kramer, M., Schulze, P. E., 'Absorption, distribution, and elimination of labeled dimethylsulfoxide in man and animals', *Annals of the New York Academy of Sciences,* 1967/141(1), 85–95

11 Kietzmann, M., Scherkl, R., Schulz, R., 'Pharmakologie der Entzündung und der Allergie', *Lehrbuch der Pharmakologie und Toxikologie für die Veterinärmedizin,* 2nd edition (Stuttgart: Enke Verlag, 2002) 318–44

12 Self, R., Casey, J. C., Swain, T., 'Origin of Methanol and Dimethyl Sulphide from Cooked Foods', *Nature,* 1963/200, 885

13 Brayton, C. F., 'Dimethyl sulfoxide (DMSO): A Review', *The Cornell Veterinarian*, 1986/76(1), 61–90

14 Martin, D., Weise, A., Niclas, H.-J., 'Das Lösungsmittel Dimethylsulfoxid', *Angewandte Chemie*, 1967/79(8), 340–57

15 Schläfer, H. L., Schaffernicht, W., 'Dimethylsulfoxyd als Lösungsmittel für anorganische Verbindungen', *Angewandte Chemie*, 1960/72(17), 618–26

16 Gaylord Chemical: 'DMSO-Sicherheitsdatenblatt gemäß 1907/2006/EG, Artikel 31, überarbeitet am. 01.05.2011 Versions-Nr: 3'

17 Sears, P. G., Lester, G. R., Dawson, L. R., 'A Study of the Conductance Behaviour of Some Uni-univalent Electrolytes in Dimethyl Sulfoxide at 25°', *Journal of Physical Chemistry*, 1956/60(10), 1433–6

18 MacGregor, W. S., 'The Chemical and Physical Properties of DMSO', *Annals of the New York Academy of Sciences*, 1967/141, 3–12

19 Walker, M., *DMSO: Nature's Healer* (New York: Avery, 1993)

20 Jacob, S. W., Herschler, R., 'Pharmacology of DMSO', *Cryobiology*, 1986/23(1), 14–27

21 Sommer, S., Tauberger, G., 'Toxikologische Untersuchungen mit Dimethylsulfoxyd', *Arzneimittel-Forschung*, 1964/14, 1050–3

22 Clinical Reports, *Annals of the New York Academy of Sciences*, 1967/141, 493

23 Ali, B. H., 'Dimethyl sulfoxide: recent pharmacological and toxicological research', *Veterinary and Human Toxicology*, 2001/43(4), 228–31

24 Wood, D. C., Wood, J., 'Pharmacologic and biochemical considerations of dimethyl sulfoxide', *Annals of the New York Academy of Sciences*, 1975/243, 7–19

25 Baptista, L., Silva, E. C. Da, Arbilla, G., 'Oxidation Mechanism of Dimethyl Sulfoxide (DMSO) by OH Radical in Liquid Phase', *Physical Chemistry Chemical Physics*, 2008/10(45), 6867–79

26 Herscu-Kluska, R., Masarwa, A., Saphier, M., Cohen, H., Meyerstein, D., 'Mechanism of the Reaction of Radicals with Peroxides and Dimethyl Sulfoxide in Aqueous Solution', *Chemical European Journal*, 2008/14(19), 5880–9

27 Chang, C. K., Albarillo, M. V., Schumer, W., 'Therapeutic effect of dimethyl sulfoxide on ICAM-1 gene expression and activation of NF-kappaB and AP-1 in septic rats', *Journal of Surgical Research*, 2001/95(2), 181–7

28 Santos, N. C., Figueira-Coelho, J., Martins-Silva, J., Saldanha, C., 'Multi-disciplinary utilization of dimethyl sulfoxide: pharmacological, cellular, and molecular aspects', *Biochemical Pharmacology*, 2003/65(7), 1035–41

29 Shealy, C. N.: 'The physiological substrate of pain', *Headache*, 1966/6(3), 101–8

30 Broadwell, R. D., Salcman, M., Kaplan, R. S., 'Morphologic effect of dimethyl sulfoxide on the blood–brain barrier', *Science*, 1982/217, 164–6

31 Saeed, S. A., Karimi, S. J., Suria, A., 'Differential effects of dimethyl sulfoxide on human platelet aggregation and arachidonic acid metabolism', *Biochemical Medicine and Metabolic Biology*, 1988/40(2), 143–50

32 Gorog, P., Kovacs, I. B., 'Antiarthritic and antithrombotic effects of topically applied dimethyl sulfoxide', *Annals of the New York Academy of Sciences*, 1975/243, 91–7

33 De la Torre, J. C., Rowed, D. W., Kawanaga, H. M., Mullan, S., 'Dimethyl sulfoxide in the treatment of experimental brain compression', *Journal of Neurosurgery*, 1973/38(3), 345–54

34 Kligman, A. M., 'Dimethyl Sulfoxide – Part 2', *The Journal of the American Medical Association*, 1965/193(11), 923–8

35 Jacob, S. W., Rosenbaum, E. E., 'Dimethylsulfoxyd: Ein Werturteil nach zweijähriger klinischer Erfahrung', *DMSO-Symposium, Vienna*, Berlin / Saladruck, 1966, 90

36 Klemm, G. M., Lindner, D., Dietz, O., Mill, J., Richter, W., 'Pharmacologic mechanism of dimethyl sulfoxide (DMSO) based on cytological studies in cattle and clinical observations in sport horses', *Monatshefte für Veterinärmedizin*, 1969/24(16), 612–18

37 Chen, D., Song, D., Wientjes, M. G., Au, J. L., 'Effect of dimethyl sulfoxide on bladder tissue penetration of intravesical paclitaxel', *Clinical Cancer Research*, 2003/9(1), 363–9

38 Douwes, R. A., van der Kolk, J. H., 'Dimethylsulfoxide (DMSO) in horses: a literature review', *Tijdschrift voor Diergeneeskunde*, 1998/123(3), 74–80

39 Ehrlich, G. E., Joseph, R., 'Dimethyl sulfoxide in scleroderma', *Pennsylvania Medical Journal*, 1965/68(12), 51–3

40 Sams, W. M. Jr., Carroll, N. V., 'Cholinesterase inhibitory property of dimethyl sulphoxide', *Nature*, 1966/212, 405

41 Perlman, R. L., Wolff, J., 'Dimethyl sulfoxide: an inhibitor of liver alcohol dehydrogenase', *Science*, 1968/160, 317–19

42 Hillidge, C. J., 'The case for dimethyl sulphoxide (DMSO) in equine practice', *Equine Veterinary Journal*, 1985/17(4), 259–61

43 Finney, J. W., Urschel, H. C. Jr., Balla, G. A., Race, George J., Jay, B. E., Pingree, H. P., Dorman, H. L., Mallams, J. T., 'Protection of the ischemic heart with DMSO alone or DMSO with hydrogen peroxide', *Annals of the New York Academy of Sciences*, 1967/141, 231–41

44 Lishner, M., Lang, R., Kedar, I., Ravid, M., 'Treatment of diabetic perforating ulcers with local DMSO', *Journal of the American Geriatrics Society,* 1985/33(1), 41–3

45 Leake, C. D., 'Dimethyl Sulfoxide', *Science,* 1966/152(7), 1646–9

46 Smith, E. R., Hadidian, Z., Mason, M. M., 'The Toxicity of Single and Repeated Dermal Applications of Dimethyl Sulfoxide', *Journal of Clinical Pharmacology,* 1968/8(5), 315–21

47 Lohs, K. von, Damerau, W., Schramm, T., ['The question of the carcinogenic action of DMSO'], *Archiv für Geschwulstforschung,* 1971/37(1), 1–3

48 David, N. A., 'The pharmacology of dimethylsulphoxide', *Annual Review of Pharmacology,* 1972/12, 353–74

49 Sulzberger, M. B., Cortese Jr., T. A., Fishman, L., Wiley, H. S., Peyakovich, P. S., 'Some effects of DMSO on human skin in vivo', *Annals of the New York Academy of Sciences,* 1967/141, 437–50

50 Brobyn, R. D., *Medical Tribune,* 1968/10, 3

51 Brobyn, R. D., 'The human toxicology of dimethylsulfoxide', *Annals of the New York Academy of Sciences,* 1975/243, 497–506

52 Kolb, K. H.: *Arzneimittel Forschung,* 1965/15, 1292

53 Wiberg, N., *Lehrbuch der Anorganischen Chemie / Holleman-Wiberg* (Berlin: W. De Gruyter, 1985), 461

54 Abdel-Rahman M. S., Gerges S. E., Alliger H., 'Toxicity of alcide', *Journal of Applied Toxicology,* 1982/2(3), 160–4

55 Imaizumi, N., Kanayama, T., Oikawa, K., 'Effect of dimethylsulfoxide as a masking agent for aqueous chlorine in the determination of oxychlorines', *Analyst,* 1995/120(7), 1983–7

56 Pies, J., *Wasserstoffsuperoxid* (Freiburg: VAK Verlag, 2004)

57 Last, W., *Krebs natürlich heilen* (Immenstadt: Mobiwell Verlag, 2010)

58 McCabe, E., *Flood your Body with Oxygen* (Carson City: Energy Publications, 2010)

59 Mutschler, E., *Arzneimittelwirkungen: Lehrbuch der Pharmakologie und Toxikologie,* 6th edition (Suttgart: Wissenschaftliche Verlagsgesellschaft, 1991)

60 Montes, M., Iglesias-Martinez, E., Penedo, F., Brandariz, I., 'Protonation constants of Procaine in different salts', *Journal of Chemical & Engineering Data,* 2008/53(7), 1514–7

61 Reuter, U., Oettmeier, R., *StK-Zeitschrift für angewandte Schmerztherapie,* 4/2000

62 *Brockhaus* 19th edition (Mannheim: Brockhaus, 1984)

63 Tucker, E. J., Carrizo, A., 'Hematoxylon dissolved in dimethyl sulfoxide used in recurrent neoplasms', *International Surgery*, 1968/49, 516–27

64 http://de.wikipedia.org/wiki/Ignaz_Semmelweis (accessed 22/0/2012)

65 Michelakis, E., et al., 'A Mitochondria-K+ Channel Axis Is Suppressed in Cancer and Its Normalization Promotes Apoptosis and Inhibits Cancer Growth', *Cancer Cell*, 2007/11(1), 37–51

66 Wenzel, U., Nickel, A., Daniel, H., 'Alpha-Lipoic acid induces apoptosis in human colon cancer cells by increasing mitochondrial respiration with a concomitant O2-*-generation', *Apoptosis*, 2005/10(2), 359–68

67 Information received personally from Emeritus Professor Siegfried Hünig, Universität Würzburg.

68 Zingerman, L. I., 'Dimethylsulfoxide in the treatment of multiple sclerosis', *Zhurnal Neuropatologii I Psikhiatrii Imeni S. S. Korsakova*, 1984/84(9), 1330–3

69 Dubner, S. J., 'How real is "Restless Legs Syndrome"?', *New York Times* (20 July 2007)

70 Woloshin S., Schwartz, L. M., 'Giving Legs to Restless Legs: A Case Study of How the Media Helps Make People Sick', http://www.plosmedicine.org/article/info:doi/10.1371/journal.pmed.0030170

71 Miranda-Tirado, R., 'Dimethylsulfoxide therapy in chronic skin ulcers', *Annals of the New York Academy of Sciences*, 1975/241, 408–11

INDEX

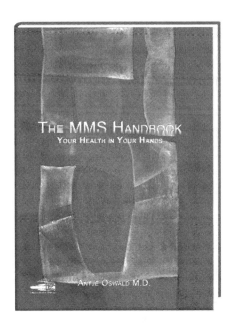

The comprehensive new reference book on MMS

Will MMS revolutionise the way many diseases are treated?

MMS – an amazing substance that consists of three atoms – can eliminate a large number of pathogens. Until now users could only draw from the experiences of a small number of brave pioneers. In this book a medical doctor addresses the subject of MMS for the first time. Dr Antje Oswald, a general practitioner in Detmold, Germany, has been intensively engaged in researching the effects of MMS and presents the fruits of that work here.

Take advantage of her knowledge and insights and discover the numerous possibilities of this phenomenal substance!

"Very readable and with plenty of depth to satisfy my thirst for details. Most importantly, it includes clear, detailed instructions for self-responsible readers on how to make use of MMS. This book has all the ingredients necessary to guarantee it a permanent place in the field of alternative medicine."
Uwe Karstädt, Alternative practitioner and author

"Thank you for the new MMS book! It has turned out fantastically and is an exciting read. Congratulations! May many people profit from it. I am delighted to recommend it to others. Great book!"
Dr Sophia Papadopoulou, General Practitioner

Paperback, 275 pages, ISBN 978-3-9815255-3-3

For more information visit www.daniel-peter-verlag.de

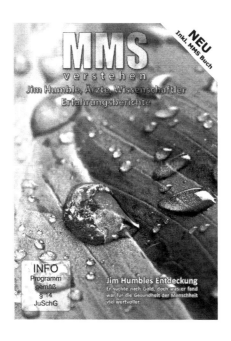

The documentary film
MMS verstehen / Understanding MMS
on DVD
fourth revised edition!

Audio in English / German / Spanish

This film imparts a deeper understanding of MMS. It features doctors, scientists and users, and you will meet in it some of the people mentioned in The MMS Handbook, such as Jim Humble, Dr John Humiston and Clara Beltrones.
The efficacy of MMS is documented using numerous first-hand reports. It is truly inspiring to learn how people have used MMS to cure serious and refractory illnesses.

Now in a fourth revised edition with:

– a 16-page booklet (in German only) which includes interesting articles on MMS, and detailed usage instructions for the most common MMS sets on the market today

– a bonus video on structured water and the surprising effect of structured water on plants.

Format DVD9. Playing time: 105 minutes. Languages: English, German, Spanish.   ISBN 978-3-9812917-0-4. Price Euros 28.00

For more information visit www.daniel-peter-verlag.de

11650450R00149

Made in the USA
Monee, IL
14 September 2019